Alternative Medicine

QUEEN ANNE HIGH
SCHOOL LIBRARY

Not for Loan

ISSUES

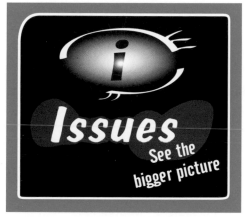

Volume 195

Series Editor

Lisa Firth

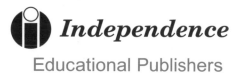 *Independence*

Educational Publishers

Cambridge

KT-449-505

First published by Independence

The Studio, High Green

Great Shelford

Cambridge CB22 5EG

England

© Independence 2010

Copyright

This book is sold subject to the condition that it shall not,
by way of trade or otherwise, be lent, resold, hired out or otherwise
circulated in any form of binding or cover other than that in which it
is published without the publisher's prior consent.

Photocopy licence

The material in this book is protected by copyright. However, the
purchaser is free to make multiple copies of particular articles for instructional
purposes for immediate use within the purchasing institution.
Making copies of the entire book is not permitted.

British Library Cataloguing in Publication Data

Alternative medicine. -- (Issues ; v. 195)

1. Alternative medicine.

I. Series II. Firth, Lisa.

615.5-dc22

ISBN-13: 978 1 86168 560 5

Printed in Great Britain

MWL Print Group Ltd

Chapter 1 Complementary Therapies

Chapter 2 The Debate

OTHER TITLES IN THE ISSUES SERIES

For more on these titles, visit: www.independence.co.uk

EXPLORING THE ISSUES

Photocopiable study guides to accompany the above publications. Each four-page A4 guide provides a variety of discussion points and other activities to suit a wide range of ability levels and interests.

A note on critical evaluation

Because the information reprinted here is from a number of different sources, readers should bear in mind the origin of the text and whether the source is likely to have a particular bias when presenting information (just as they would if undertaking their own research). It is hoped that, as you read about the many aspects of the issues explored in this book, you will critically evaluate the information presented. It is important that you decide whether you are being presented with facts or opinions. Does the writer give a biased or an unbiased report? If an opinion is being expressed, do you agree with the writer?

Alternative Medicine offers a useful starting point for those who need convenient access to information about the many issues involved. However, it is only a starting point. Following each article is a URL to the relevant organisation's website, which you may wish to visit for further information.

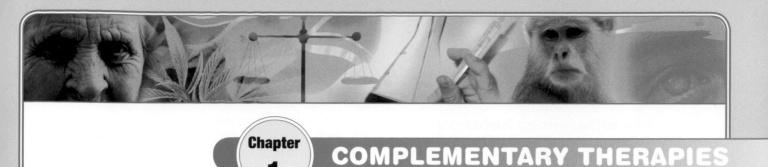

An introduction to complementary therapy

Information from Arthritis Research UK.

What is complementary and alternative medicine?

Complementary and alternative medicine includes a wide range of therapies and practices that are outside the mainstream of medicine.

⇨ Complementary medicine uses therapies that work alongside conventional medicine.

⇨ Alternative medicine includes treatments that are not currently considered part of evidence-based Western medicine.

More and more health professionals such as doctors, nurses and physiotherapists use various kinds of complementary and alternative medicine

The distinction between alternative and complementary medicine isn't clear cut. For this reason, the term complementary and alternative medicine (or CAM) is now widely used to include both approaches. Integrated medicine means that conventional, complementary and alternative therapies are brought together in the same place.

More and more health professionals such as doctors, nurses and physiotherapists use various kinds of complementary and alternative medicine, including acupuncture, homeopathy, manipulation and aromatherapy. As research continues, some of these treatments may become more recognised.

Complementary and alternative therapists

There are two main groups of complementary and alternative therapists: those who are legally registered and those who are not.

⇨ Osteopaths and chiropractors are legally recognised professionals just like doctors, nurses and physiotherapists.

  ↳ Their training is regulated by a body set up by the Government.

  ↳ They must be insured.

  ↳ They can be struck off and prevented from practising if they are incompetent or unethical.

⇨ The Government is considering whether to legally register herbalists, acupuncturists and traditional Chinese medicine practitioners. A decision is expected in 2010, but at the time of writing they were not legally registered.

⇨ Many other complementary and alternative therapists are not legally registered (even if they describe themselves as registered). Many of these therapists are good, but it is difficult to be sure.

If you use complementary and alternative medicine, it is important that you discuss this with your doctor and healthcare team and don't suddenly stop your conventional medicine. You should be suspicious of any complementary and alternative medicine practitioner who advises you to do so.

What should you look for when choosing a therapist?

There are some guidelines that patients should consider when sourcing a complementary or alternative therapist.

If you consult a complementary and alternative medicine practitioner, he or she should:

⇨ have an agreed code of ethics;

⇨ be insured in case something goes wrong with your treatment;

⇨ be a member of an organisation that promotes self-regulation and does not make unreasonable claims about their treatments.

A new independent self-regulatory body for complementary therapies, supported by the Government, the Complementary and Natural Healthcare Council (CNHC), was set up in 2008. It is possible to find a registered therapist from this body.

ARTHRITIS RESEARCH UK

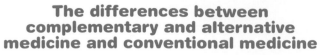

The differences between complementary and alternative medicine and conventional medicine

This section looks at the differences between conventional medicine and alternative or complementary therapies.

Complementary and alternative medicine

The ways in which complementary and alternative therapies are thought to work are diverse, although many are based on the idea of self-healing.

⇨ Complementary and alternative medicine tends to be holistic, i.e. they treat the whole person, not just the symptoms of a disease.

⇨ This usually requires more lifestyle changes (i.e. diet, exercise and positive thinking) than conventional treatments. This may be a key to their continuing success with those who have tried them.

⇨ Wellness comes from a balance between the body, mind and the environment.

⇨ Each person is treated as a unique individual who has his or her own particular make-up, is subject to a unique combination of stresses, lives in a unique environment, and has his or her own healing mechanisms to recover from illness.

⇨ Many forms of complementary and alternative medicine aim to stimulate or enable the body's ability to heal itself.

⇨ Many complementary and alternative therapies require the individual's active participation in the treatment.

Conventional medicine

Conventional medicine researches and tries to understand and correct the underlying abnormalities that cause the disease. In many instances the underlying abnormalities are not fully understood. However, there have been major advances, especially in rheumatoid arthritis, in recent years, with much of the research being funded by Arthritis Research UK. Conventional medicine is often criticised for treating the disease and not the individual, requiring the patient to accept the diagnosis and treatment. It may be due to the influence of complementary and alternative medicine, but conventional medicine is increasingly recognising the importance of the patient's involvement and choice in their treatment.

Are complementary and alternative therapies safe to use?

Safety is very important to people who use complementary and alternative therapies. Many turn to complementary and alternative medicine because they have suffered side-effects from conventional treatment. It is difficult to generalise, but generally speaking complementary and alternative therapies are relatively safe.

You should, however, always discuss their use with your doctor before starting treatment as there are some risks associated with specific therapies. For instance:

⇨ Infectious diseases can be transmitted by acupuncture needles, which can be avoided if single-use needles are used.

⇨ A number of herbal therapies may be associated with significant side-effects:

  ↳ Echinacea may cause rashes.

  ↳ St John's wort may interact with other drugs (for example warfarin, requiring adjustment of the dose) or with the contraceptive pill, which may stop working and so an alternative means of contraception should be used, and other drugs.

  ↳ Some natural therapies such as natural hormone replacement therapy (HRT) contain plant oestrogens that may cause irregular menstrual bleeding.

  ↳ There are some reports of the wrong or contaminated herbs being used in herbal mixtures and causing serious side-effects.

In many cases the risks associated with complementary and alternative therapies are associated more with the therapist than the therapy – for instance a trained acupuncturist would never reuse needles, and a trained herbalist will be aware of the possible risks.

⇨ The above information is reprinted with kind permission from Arthritis Research UK. Visit www.arthritisresearchuk.org for more information.

© Arthritis Research UK

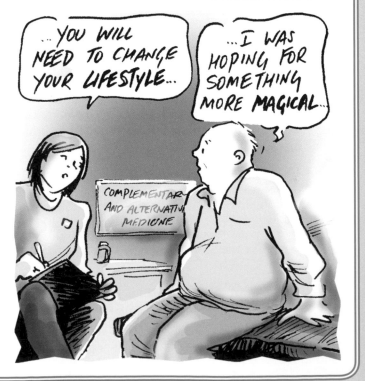

ARTHRITIS RESEARCH UK

Complementary and alternative medicine

Information from Patient UK.

Complementary and alternative medicine (CAM) includes a group of diverse medical and healthcare systems, practices and products that are not generally considered part of conventional medicine. Complementary medicine is generally regarded as a complementary treatment that is used alongside conventional medicine whereas alternative medicine is regarded as a treatment used in place of conventional medicine.

CAM may be practised by those with a medical qualification, as is often the case with acupuncture or homeopathy. They may also be practised by those with another relevant qualification such as physiotherapy, as may be the case with manipulation. However, patients should be alerted to practitioners who have no specific training or registration in CAM.

A good reason for registration of all CAM practitioners is to ascertain that they are appropriately trained and that they also comply with certain ethical standards and undergo some form of peer review and continued professional development.

There has been considerable interest in CAM, with a House of Lords Select Committee Report in November 2000 and a subcommittee of the Royal College of Physicians set up to examine certain aspects. They reported in *Clinical Medicine* in 2003.

The House of Lords Select Committee was very keen that there should be professional standards, registration and accountability in all aspects of CAM. The acupuncture profession will be statutorily regulated by 2010. Osteopathy is regulated by the General Osteopathic Council. Chiropractic is regulated by the General Chiropractic Council.

Popularity of complementary and alternative medicine

In the UK, research published in 2001 showed that 47% of people have used CAM at some time in their lives and 10% use some form of CAM each year. Users tend to be older and female. Over 90% is purchased outside of the NHS. At least 10% of hospital physicians are also thought to use CAM as part of their clinical practice. A survey conducted in 2001 estimated that one in two practices in England now offer their patients some access to CAM.

A report in the *Lancet* in 2007 stated that about 13,000 patients were treated at the five (now four) homeopathic hospitals in the UK each year; 14.5% of the population say that they trust homeopathy and £38 million is spent on homeopathy each year in the UK. Of the various forms of CAM, acupuncture is amongst the most popular. Approximately three million people undergo acupuncture treatment in the UK each year.

Examples of complementary and alternative medicine practices

There are a great many approaches that may be classified as CAM. There are also activities such as yoga and tai chi and various diets where health benefits are claimed and some may regard them as CAM.

Separate articles on the Patient UK website discuss:

⇨ Acupuncture.

⇨ Homeopathy.

⇨ Back Manipulation (Osteopathy and Chiropractic).

⇨ Aromatherapy.

⇨ Reflexology.

Other examples of CAM include:

⇨ Herbal remedies.

⇨ Hypnosis.

⇨ Diets, including the 'macrobiotic diet'.

⇨ Chelation therapy.

⇨ Faith healing.

Herbal remedies

The medicinal properties of herbs have been exploited for many centuries. The druids and the ancient Egyptians are amongst the best-known exponents of herbal medicine. Nicholas Culpeper's work in the 17th century was seminal. Bearing in mind the origins of such drugs as digoxin, aspirin, quinine and penicillin, it would be surprising if other plants or micro-organisms did not also offer therapeutic potential. However, it would also be surprising if they did not have adverse effects. If digoxin had been discovered recently, it may not have received a product licence, as the ratio of toxic to therapeutic dose is too low.

The concern is that many herbal remedies that are for sale have not been thoroughly tested for efficacy, toxicity, drug interactions and teratogenicity. In addition there are often problems of variation in potency between batches, and correct doses are not carefully established.

The problem with herbal remedies is that they may well have pharmacological properties. As such, they can be expected to have some of the same problems as licensed drugs, including adverse effects. Ideally, before any herbal remedy is allowed to be marketed, there are a number of questions

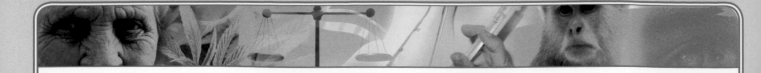

that should be answered, as for conventional medicines:

⇨ Is potency reliable or is there marked variation between batches?

⇨ Is it effective? This needs double-blind randomised controlled trials of appropriate sizes.

⇨ What is the appropriate dose?

⇨ What is the toxic dose?

⇨ What is the adverse effect profile?

⇨ What interactions are there with other drugs that may commonly be used simultaneously?

⇨ Is it teratogenic? If that question cannot be answered, there must be warnings about pregnancy.

The Medicines and Healthcare products Regulatory Agency (MHRA) is the government agency which is responsible for ensuring that medicines and medical devices work, and are acceptably safe. They say that the current weak regulation of herbal remedies in the UK has led to specific safety concerns. There are three regulatory routes by which a herbal remedy can reach consumers:

1 As unlicensed herbal remedies – there are no specific standards of safety and quality and so standards can vary widely. They are not required to be sold with product information for consumers to use them safely, such as safety warnings and contra-indications. This situation is not ideal and by April 2011 all manufactured herbal medicines will be required to have either a traditional herbal registration or a product licence (see below).

2 As registered traditional herbal medicines – the Traditional Herbal Medicines Registration Scheme (THMRS) began on 30th October 2005. Products have to meet specific standards of safety and quality. They have to be accompanied by agreed indications, based on traditional usage, and systematic patient information allowing the safe use of the product. There is a nine-digit registration number starting with the letters 'THR' on the container or packaging.

3 As licensed herbal medicines – some herbal medicines in the UK hold a product licence or marketing authorisation, as any other medicine. Such medicines are required to demonstrate safety, quality and efficacy and be accompanied by information for safe usage. There is a nine-number product licence (PL) number on the container or packaging, prefixed by the letters 'PL'.

The MHRA website also provides a list of herbal ingredients which are prohibited or restricted in medicines.

There is a separate article on the Patient UK website on St John's wort, which is one of the best researched of all the various herbal remedies.

Hypnosis

Hypnosis may be practised by medically-qualified people, clinical psychologists or those without healthcare qualifications. Hypnosis must be used with skill and care, as adverse events, including the implantation of false memories, may occur. The British Society of Clinical Hypnosis can help in finding a registered practitioner. Both competence and ethics are essential.

Conditions amenable to treatment include:

⇨ Smoking cessation.

⇨ Nail biting.

⇨ Weight control.

⇨ Healthy eating.

⇨ Sports performance.

⇨ Exam nerves.

⇨ Irrational fears and phobias.

⇨ Stress management.

⇨ Compulsive behaviour.

⇨ Anxiety and panic attacks.

⇨ Stress-related stomach and digestive problems.

⇨ Childbirth.

⇨ Some skin problems.

⇨ Pain control.

⇨ Stress-related high blood pressure.

⇨ Self-confidence.

⇨ Compulsions and compulsive behaviour.

⇨ Some sexual problems.

There have been a number of systematic reviews, including Cochrane reviews of the various topics.

Diets

There is no doubt that diet is very important and that it can have a profound influence on arterial disease and cancer. However, there is concern over 'fad' and 'trendy' diets of unproven value that may be inadequate in terms of effective nutrition, especially in children.

The aim of the macrobiotic diet is to avoid foods containing toxins. It is a completely vegan diet and no dairy products or meats are allowed. Macrobiotic diets have become popular with people who have cancer, who believe that it can help them fight their cancer and lead to a cure. However, there is no scientific evidence to prove that a macrobiotic diet can treat or cure cancer or any other disease.

Some research shows that macrobiotic diets may improve health in some people as long as they are not followed to an extreme. This may be because of an increase in

PATIENT UK

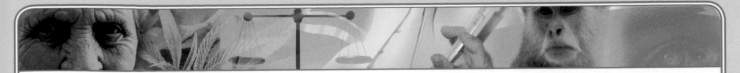

fruit and vegetable intake and a reduction in fat, sugar and salt intake. However, a 'normal' diet can also allow this. There is concern that for some people, following a macrobiotic diet can have serious, harmful effects such as nutrient deficiencies and weight loss. They are also very expensive.

Chelation therapy

Chelation therapy is the use of chelating agents – usually the man-made amino acid ethylene diamine tetra-acetic acid (EDTA) – to remove heavy metals from the body. It is of proven value in Wilson's disease, haemochromatosis and heavy metal poisoning (including lead and mercury). However, it has also been promoted by some for the treatment of other disorders, including arterial disease, Alzheimer's disease and autism.

The basis for its use in arterial disease is the belief that it also chelates calcium, one of the components of atherosclerotic plaques. The American Heart Association has spoken out against the use of chelation therapy in arterial disease. It has concluded that the benefits claimed for this form of therapy aren't scientifically proven, and so they therefore do not recommend its use.

Faith healing

Faith healing is not new. It is well documented in both the Old Testament (Second Book of Kings, chapter 5) and New Testament (Gospel of Luke, chapter 8, verses 26 to 56) of the Bible, along with the observation that it is only effective where there is absolute faith. There are still charismatic preachers who carry out 'faith' healing in which people come to the front and publicly discard the wheelchairs that they have allegedly depended upon for many years.

Many churches, including traditionally reserved sections of the Church of England, have taken to 'healing services' but they are not to be confused with the hysteria of the charismatic performances. They do not try to portray their role as a substitute for medical care but more as an adjunct. However, much as we may try to be holistic, patients may have spiritual needs that are not within our remit. This is where religious organisations can help. They may be beneficial in helping the person to live in peace with his disease, and perhaps we should not always equate 'healing' with 'cure'.

Reasons for using complementary and alternative medicine

It is important to try to understand someone's motivation for using CAM. There may be many reasons that they may choose it. Talk to patients and find out what they are doing and why.

For example, many people have the belief that CAM techniques are 'natural' when compared to conventional medicine. There is an implication that 'natural' means invariably effective and invariably safe. However, as discussed above in the 'Herbal remedies' section, considering the array of toxins in nature, anything that is natural is not invariably safe. Interestingly, there are well-documented cases of 'herbal remedies' for childhood eczema that have been found to contain potent topical corticosteroids.

Another reason why patients may choose CAM is that they receive more time, empathy and emotional support from an alternative therapist. There may also be a spiritual component that they like. However, this shouldn't be confused with efficacy of a treatment. They may feel that their own doctor has little time or understanding for their problems. This is one reason why an holistic approach is important for all doctors.

Patients may also turn to CAM when they feel that conventional medicine has 'let them down'. For example, people with eczema, psoriasis or irritable bowel syndrome may wish to take control of their disease where they feel that conventional medicine has failed to cure them. Therapies that encourage relaxation may be useful in these conditions. If a patient is taking the usual medication for irritable bowel syndrome but also having some aromatherapy, this may well be beneficial and is unlikely to do harm.

On the other hand, there may be cases where patients may be put at risk when using CAM: for example, if parents have decided that their children should have homeopathic vaccines. Explain to them that these vaccines do not induce an antibody response against the diseases and that the Faculty of Homeopathy says that all children should have conventional vaccines.

Conclusion

Professor Ernst from Exeter University is seen by many in the CAM community as being antagonistic to their cause. This he denies. He says that he is trying to validate CAM by putting it on the same evidence base as conventional medicine.

There is some evidence that CAM may work for certain conditions but, for many conditions for which it is currently used, the evidence is of poor quality and it is impossible to draw a firm conclusion about its effectiveness. However, we must remember that this is not the same as evidence of lack of efficacy. More research is needed in this area.

CAM does appeal to patients. We, as doctors, should help our patients to make informed decisions about their healthcare. We must provide them with the evidence about CAM to aid their empowerment and decision-making process.

Last updated: 1 September 2009

⇨ Information from Patient UK. Visit www.patient.co.uk for more.

© EMIS 2010 as distributed at www.patient.co.uk/ doctor/Alternative-and-Holistic-Medicine.htm, used with permission

PATIENT UK

Why people use complementary or alternative therapies

Information from Cancer Research UK.

Who uses complementary therapies?

In the UK, up to one-third of people with cancer (33%) use some sort of complementary therapy at some time during their illness. For some types of cancer, such as breast cancer, the number of people using complementary therapies is even higher at almost half (50%).

There is no evidence to suggest that any type of complementary therapy prevents or cures cancer. But people are very interested in using complementary therapies for many reasons, including those mentioned in this article. For some therapies there is currently very little research evidence to show that they help with certain symptoms – for example, pain or hot flushes. But more reliable research studies are being carried out and we are beginning to collect evidence for some types of therapy. For example, improved quality of life following mindfulness-based stress reduction, and reduced chemotherapy-related nausea in people who have acupuncture.

In the UK, up to one-third of people with cancer (33%) use some sort of complementary therapy at some time during their illness

Despite the lack of evidence for many types of complementary therapy, many people with cancer say they gain a lot of benefit from using them.

Using therapies to help you feel better

People often use complementary therapies to help them feel better and cope with having cancer and treatment. How you feel plays a part in how you cope with having cancer. Many complementary therapies concentrate on boosting relaxation and reducing stress. They may help to calm your emotions, relieve anxiety and increase your general sense of health and well-being. Many doctors and researchers are getting more interested in the idea that positive emotions can improve your health.

Reducing symptoms or side-effects

There is increasing evidence that certain complementary therapies can help to control some of the symptoms and side-effects of cancer and treatments. For example, acupuncture can help to relieve sickness caused by some chemotherapy drugs and a sore mouth caused by treatment for head and neck cancer. It can also help to relieve pain after surgery to remove lymph nodes in the neck. CancerHelp UK has detailed information about acupuncture.

Feeling more in control

When you are having conventional cancer treatment, it may sometimes feel as though your doctor makes all the decisions about your treatment. It can begin to feel like you don't have much control over what happens to you. Many people say that complementary therapies allow them to take a more active role in their treatment and recovery. You decide which therapy to use and how often you use it. Complementary therapies may also help people to feel more in control of their feelings and emotions.

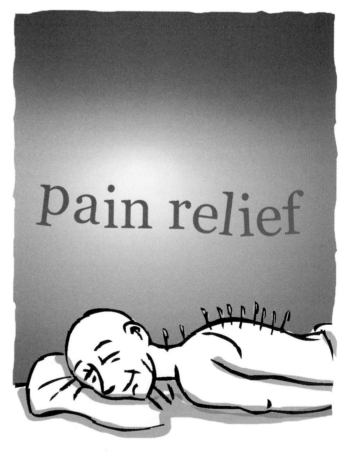

pain relief

CANCER RESEARCH UK

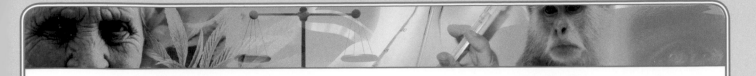

One patient who used complementary therapies alongside chemotherapy and radiotherapy said:

'I turn up for my appointment and someone injects the drugs into me, or shines radiation beams at me. Although I know all the staff care, I sometimes go away feeling very alone and not in control of my situation. But after a massage I feel less alone and more able to cope with things.'

'Natural and healing therapies'

Many patients use complementary therapies because they like the idea that they seem 'non-toxic and natural'. They also appeal to people because many therapies treat the 'whole person', not just a part of you. This is known as 'holistic healthcare'. This means that therapists look at you as a whole person, including your emotional and psychological needs, not just your physical ones.

Although many complementary therapies are 'natural' it doesn't necessarily mean they can't cause harm. Some herbal remedies may cause side effects or interfere with your conventional treatments. CancerHelp UK has detailed information about the safety of complementary and alternative therapies.

Comfort from 'touch, talk and time'

Another reason people may use complementary therapies is because they get a lot of comfort and satisfaction from the 'touch, talk and time' that a complementary therapist usually offers. Doctors' schedules are often so busy that they don't have the time they need to deal with patients' emotional and psychological needs. And they may not have had the necessary training to give that kind of care.

A skilled and caring aromatherapist, for example, has the time to make you feel cared for and so may help improve your quality of life. So a good complementary therapist can often play a very supportive role during cancer treatment and recovery.

Staying positive

Having a positive outlook is an important part of coping with cancer for most people. Even if your doctor tells you that your cancer might be difficult to cure, of course you will still want and hope for a cure. This is normal and often a very important part of coping with having cancer. Some people use complementary therapies as a way of helping themselves feel positive and hopeful for the future.

Boosting your immune system

Some people believe that certain complementary therapies can boost their immune system and help fight their cancer. But there is very little scientific evidence to back this up. Some clinical trials are looking at how certain complementary therapies might affect your immune system.

Looking for a cure

Some people may believe that specific alternative therapies may help control or cure their cancer if they are used instead of conventional cancer treatment. And there are people who promote therapies in this way. Using an alternative cancer treatment can become more important to people with advanced cancer if their conventional treatment is no longer controlling the cancer. Understandably they may feel very anxious and desperate and hope that alternative therapies may save their life or help them live longer.

There is no scientific evidence to prove that any type of alternative therapy can help to control or cure cancer. Some alternative therapies are unsafe and may cause serious side effects. CancerHelp UK has detailed information about the safety of complementary and alternative therapies.

⇨ Taken from CancerHelp UK, the patient information website of Cancer Research UK: www.cancerhelp.org.uk

© Cancer Research UK

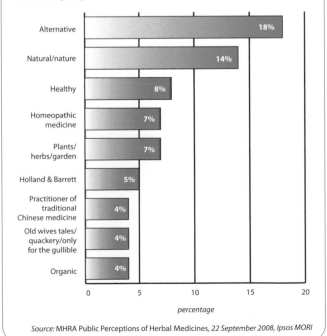

Respondents were asked 'What words or phrases come to mind when I say "herbal medicines"?'

This graph gives only responses specified by 4% or more of respondents. Details of other responses can be found in the topline results for this survey at this URL: http://www.ipsos-mori.com/Assets/Docs/Polls/public-perceptions-of-herbal-medicines-topline.pdf

	percentage
Alternative	18%
Natural/nature	14%
Healthy	8%
Homeopathic medicine	7%
Plants/herbs/garden	7%
Holland & Barrett	5%
Practitioner of traditional Chinese medicine	4%
Old wives tales/quackery/only for the gullible	4%
Organic	4%

Source: MHRA Public Perceptions of Herbal Medicines, 22 September 2008, Ipsos MORI

Alternative antidotes

Information from YouGov.

By Sara Lofberg

A new report from YouGov SixthSense highlighting UK pharmaceutical spending habits reveals that the quick and convenient low-budget fix wins out when it comes to buying non-prescribed medicinal products. 'Alternative' and herbal remedies are also popular, especially among women.

The larger, non-prescriptive medicinal brands are seen as 'expensive' by 28% of targeted UK consumers, but not necessarily more effective. Accordingly, 39% say that when buying painkillers such as paracetamol or ibuprofen they would opt for a lower-priced brand. In comparison, only 26% say they would buy a 'well-known brand'.

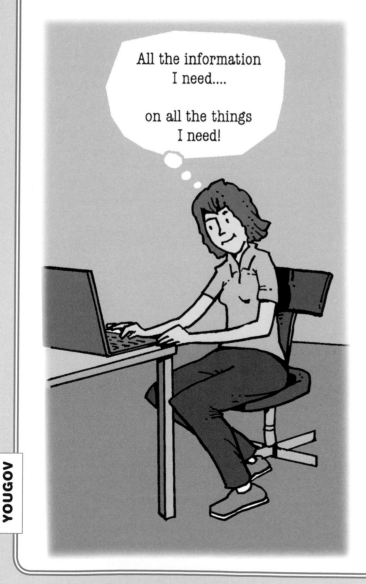

All the information I need....

on all the things I need!

Moreover, consumers prefer to buy their non-prescriptive drugs at the supermarket (a substantial 78% prefer this) compared to other sources, such as chemists' or over the Internet. Only 2% of UK consumers currently buy most of their medicines or healthcare treatments online, and only 11% say that they buy a 'few' products in this way; 66% say they have never bought medicine online and are 'unlikely to ever do so'.

James McCoy, Research Director of YouGov SixthSense, explains, 'People are quite *laissez-faire* when it comes to the purchasing of non-prescribed pharmaceutical products. Brand loyalty is generally low and we have no qualms with going for the quickest, cheapest and most convenient route to pain relief. These trends would appear to account for the popularity of supermarkets as a place of purchase for these items.'

Herbal help

But it's a different story when it comes to specifically herbal and 'alternative' remedies. Customers go beyond the store shelves and turn to online shopping when seeking treatments like St John's wort, vitamin supplements and homeopathic products.

Indeed, 18% of respondents say they have bought some kind of herbal remedy online in the past 12 months, while homeopathic treatments, multivitamins and Omega 3 tablets constitute a staggering 41% of medicines respondents have bought via the Internet in the same time period. There's a clear gender gap though: 75% of those who have used homeopathic/alternative remedies in the last 12 months are women, as are 81% of those who say they currently have homeopathic/alternative remedies in their medicine cabinet.

McCoy continues, 'A growth in online retailing in non-prescribed products might lead to a larger payoff for wholesalers of alternative medicines; with less personal interaction with qualified pharmacists, consumers may be willing to follow their own research and take a chance on alternative medicines.'

Indeed, herbal and alternative treatments are relatively well credited amongst UK consumers as one in four respondents believes that they are effective in treating or preventing minor ailments, despite only one in ten people consulting a pharmacist before making a non-prescription purchase.

9 July 2010

⇨ The above information is reprinted with kind permission from YouGov. Visit www.yougov.com for more information.

© YouGov

YOUGOV

Traditional medicine: definitions

The following terms are extracted from the General Guidelines for Methodologies on Research and Evaluation of Traditional Medicine.

Traditional medicine

Traditional medicine is the sum total of the knowledge, skills and practices based on the theories, beliefs, and experiences indigenous to different cultures, whether explicable or not, used in the maintenance of health as well as in the prevention, diagnosis, improvement or treatment of physical and mental illness.

Complementary/alternative medicine (CAM)

The terms 'complementary medicine' or 'alternative medicine' are used interchangeably with traditional medicine in some countries. They refer to a broad set of healthcare practices that are not part of that country's own tradition and are not integrated into the dominant healthcare system.

Herbal medicines

Herbal medicines include herbs, herbal materials, herbal preparations and finished herbal products, that contain as active ingredients parts of plants, or other plant materials, or combinations.

⇨ Herbs: crude plant material such as leaves, flowers, fruit, seed, stems, wood, bark, roots, rhizomes or other plant parts, which may be entire, fragmented or powdered.

⇨ Herbal materials: in addition to herbs, fresh juices, gums, fixed oils, essential oils, resins and dry powders of herbs. In some countries, these materials may be processed by various local procedures, such as steaming, roasting, or stir-baking with honey, alcoholic beverages or other materials.

⇨ Herbal preparations: the basis for finished herbal products and may include comminuted or powdered herbal materials, or extracts, tinctures and fatty oils of herbal materials. They are produced by extraction, fractionation, purification, concentration, or other physical or biological processes. They also include preparations made by steeping or heating herbal materials in alcoholic beverages and/or honey, or in other materials.

⇨ Finished herbal products: herbal preparations made from one or more herbs. If more than one herb is used, the term 'mixture herbal product' can also be used. Finished herbal products and mixture herbal products may contain excipients in addition to the active ingredients. However, finished products or mixture products to which chemically defined active substances have been added, including synthetic compounds and/or isolated constituents from herbal materials, are not considered to be herbal.

Traditional use of herbal medicines

Traditional use of herbal medicines refers to the long historical use of these medicines. Their use is well established and widely acknowledged to be safe and effective, and may be accepted by national authorities.

Traditional use of herbal medicines refers to the long historical use of these medicines. Their use is well established and widely acknowledged to be safe and effective

---

Therapeutic activity

Therapeutic activity refers to the successful prevention, diagnosis and treatment of physical and mental illnesses; improvement of symptoms of illnesses; as well as beneficial alteration or regulation of the physical and mental status of the body.

Active ingredients

Active ingredients refer to ingredients of herbal medicines with therapeutic activity. In herbal medicines where the active ingredients have been identified, the preparation of these medicines should be standardised to contain a defined amount of the active ingredients, if adequate analytical methods are available. In cases where it is not possible to identify the active ingredients, the whole herbal medicine may be considered as one active ingredient.

⇨ The above information is reprinted with kind permission from the World Health Organization. Visit www.who.int for more information.

© World Health Organization

WORLD HEALTH ORGANIZATION

Herbal and traditional medicine

Information from the European Herbal and Traditional Medicine Practitioners Association.

EUROPEAN HERBAL AND TRADITIONAL MEDICINE PRACTITIONERS ASSOCIATION

Herbal medicine is among the most ancient forms of treatment known and the medicinal use of plants is common to all cultures and peoples of the world. The Egyptian *Ebers Papyrus*, dating back to 1500 BCE, describes more than 700 herbal remedies including aloes, caraway seeds, castor oil and squill. A medical manuscript, *Wu Shi Er Ming Fang*, dating from the 2nd century BCE listing some 224 herbal medicines was discovered in 1973 in a tomb at Ma Huang Dui in Hunan Province, China. The Atharva Veda dating from about 1200 BCE is recognised as a major source book laying down the precepts of Ayurveda, the ancient system of medicine from India. There was significant exchange of herbal knowledge in the ancient world. Hippocrates, 'the father of medicine', was tutored by Egyptian priest doctors. Dioscorides, a Greek doctor attached to the Roman armies of Claudius and Nero, compiled ancient and contemporary herbal knowledge in his famous herbal *De Materia Medica* that for more than 13 centuries remained one of the principal medical textbooks throughout the civilised world. The Greek herbal achieved its final form in the work of Claudius Galen who was physician to the Roman Emperor, Marcus Aurelius.

The medicine of medieval Europe was significantly advanced by herbal skills brought back to Europe by the Crusaders, who learnt their medicine from their Arab adversaries who had themselves synthesised the knowledge of ancient Greek and Persian medicine.

For many centuries plant remedies were the main medicines used to treat disease throughout Europe and many famous herbals were published in English in the 16th and 17th centuries. Some, like those of Culpeper and Gerard, are still well-known today. However, with the dawn of the scientific age came the slow decline of plant-based medicine accelerated by the widespread introduction in the 18th century of minerals and metal-based remedies into medicine such as arsenic, antimony, lead, mercury, copper, tin and gold. John Waller commented on this trend in his *British Domestic Herbal*, published in 1822:

'Advantages have accrued to medicine from chemical preparations. It is nevertheless a melancholy truth that the health of thousands and the lives of not a few are yearly sacrificed to the rage for preparations of mercury, arsenic and almost every deleterious mineral under heaven. So far has this rage for poisonous drugs gained ground that scarcely any article from the plant kingdom is thought worthy to enter into the prescription of a modern physician that is not recognised for a dangerous and active poison; hence the daily use of aconite, hemlock, henbane, etc.'

With the discovery of antibiotics, corticosteroids and other major modern drugs, the vast majority of herbal remedies used by doctors for many centuries became relegated to mere footnotes in the official pharmacopoeias. They remained, however, the remedies of choice of UK herbalists and the practitioners of other herbal traditions that have recently taken root in Britain, all of whom have continued these forms of traditional medicine into modern times.

⇨ The above information is reprinted with kind permission from the European Herbal and Traditional Medicine Practitioners Association. Visit http://ehtpa.eu for more information.

© European Herbal and Traditional Medicine Practitioners Association

Herbal medicine

If the laboratory drugs don't work, or you're keen to explore the options, you might consider the natural alternative. Herbal remedies may be easily available, but do they really work?

What is it?

Herbal medicines are plant-based remedies, and have been in use since early civilisation in many different forms. Today, they are commonly available as tablets, tinctures, powders, teas, food supplements and extracts. Herbal medicine also plays a central role in other forms of complementary therapy, such as homeopathy, naturotherapy and also traditional Chinese medicine (which is underpinned by a philosophy that good health comes from balance – known as yin and yang) and Ayurvedic medicine (a herbal-based therapy which is based on an Indian belief system).

Herbal medicines are plant-based remedies, and have been in use since early civilisation in many different forms

How does it work?

Herbalists believe that the delicate chemical make-up of each plant- or herb-based product contains certain healing properties. Unlike conventional medicine, however, no attempt is made to isolate and extract such elements. Instead, the belief is that the entire plant or herb should be used in order to preserve the healing properties. It's worth noting that some conventional medicines are derived from herbalism, such as aspirin (from willow bark) and morphine (from poppies).

What are the benefits?

Some herbal medicines have been tested, with proven results. For example, St John's wort is recognised in the treatment of mild depression, garlic is known to reduce blood cholesterol levels, and ginger is often used to relieve feelings of nausea. Other popular herbal remedies include Echinacea to help ease cold symptoms and peppermint oil in the treatment of Irritable Bowel Syndrome. People with allergies, sleep disorders and skin conditions also commonly turn to herbalism for treatment. Like any medicine, however, herbal products have the potential to produce unwanted reactions, and should be used with care. If in doubt, consult your doctor (GP).

Where's the proof?

It is a fact that many plants contain chemical compounds that can have an effect on the body. While many herbal products have been scientifically proven to have a beneficial impact on health, many remain untested or even questionable in nature. The key is to be sure that what you're taking is safe for your health, and only your doctor can address that.

Getting treatment

NHS herbal medicine is now available, in a very limited capacity, and much also depends on your doctor's view of complementary therapies. You can also check out the website for the National Institute of Medical Herbalists which offers an online facility to find a herbalist in your area.

Case study – Helena, 17

Recently I went to see the herbalist with a variety of problems, which are all (more or less) caused by stress. She went through my health history, and then she took my pulse and blood pressure. Once this was done, she created a blend of herbal tinctures for me to take twice a day for a month, and gave me a food diary to fill out. She then asked me to come back in a month's time to see how I got on. She also recommended that I eat some different foods (more nuts, and leafy greens), and encouraged me to drink more herbal teas, such as peppermint for my digestion and chamomile for the stress. So far, I've been far more chilled out, but it is still early days. I'd like to see how I feel by the end of the month.

If you're considering a complementary treatment or therapy for any medical condition, always consult your doctor (GP) first. This is to make sure it doesn't conflict with any existing course of treatment you may be taking, and also to check it won't have a negative impact on your health.

⇨ The above information is reprinted with kind permission from TheSite. Visit their website at www.thesite.org for more information.

© TheSite.org

THESITE.ORG

Just how safe are herbal medicines?

While many of us believe that 'herbal' is synonymous with 'safe', herbal remedies can in fact be deadly, says Tammy Cohen.

Herbal remedies made from plant leaves, bark, berries, flowers and roots have been used to heal illnesses, diseases and psychological disorders for centuries. Today, with the ease of the Internet, you can self-diagnose, order next-day delivery, and even learn how to make your own. Last year three million Britons took herbal remedies to treat everything from fever to joint pain.

But renewed debate about the safety of these remedies was sparked last week following the news of an EU crackdown on herbalists and Chinese medicine practitioners who operate unregulated at present. Under the new law, from 2011 sales of all herbal remedies except for a small number of products for minor ailments will also be banned. Regulators warn that many of us believe that 'herbal' is synonymous with 'safe', whereas herbal remedies can be deadly.

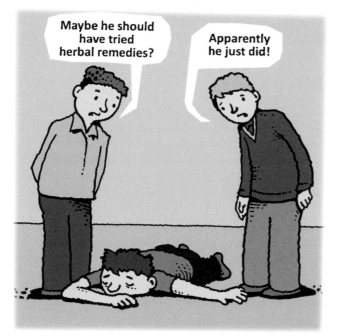

'Research we conducted last year found a significant proportion of people believed "herbal" means "benign",' says Richard Woodfield, Head of Herbal Policy at the Medicines and Healthcare products Regulatory Agency (MHRA). 'That means people are more liable to self-medicate, and to neglect to inform their doctors, even though there's a risk that the herbal remedy will react with any prescription drugs. They're also more vulnerable to fraudulent, even criminal operators who put products out which are heavily adulterated with dangerous pharmaceuticals.'

The actress Sophie Winkleman is reported to have taken aconite, or monkshood, found in some 'herbal Valium' last month to calm her nerves prior to her wedding to Freddie Windsor.

The plant, while relatively harmless in licensed homeopathic remedies in which it is rigorously diluted, can be extremely dangerous in herbal remedies, even lethal.

'If you were to buy aconite root, which is banned from licensed herbal products in the UK, but can still be found in products bought over the Internet, and make yourself a herbal tea with it, you'd be dead within five minutes,' says Dr Linda Anderson, Pharmaceutical Assessor of the MHRA.

Last year, scientists at Boston University found that a fifth of Ayurvedic medicines – popular traditional Indian herbal remedies – bought over the Internet contained dangerous levels of lead, mercury or arsenic, which could cause stomach pains, vomiting or liver problems.

Earlier this year, herbal arthritis remedies came under scrutiny when looked at as part of the Arthritis Research Campaign's (ARC) study of complementary therapies. 'Not only did we find that in two-thirds of cases, there was no evidence they actually worked, but one Chinese remedy used to combat rheumatoid arthritis – Thunder God Vine – was also reported to be extremely poisonous if not extracted properly,' says ARC spokeswoman Jane Tadman.

Menopause remedies also came under fire after a study reported in the *Drugs and Therapeutics Bulletin*, a journal that reviews medical treatment, found no evidence they actually worked. Gynaecologist Heather Curry of the British Menopause Society says: 'Our feeling is that there isn't enough scientific evidence either on effectiveness or safety.' A German study last year found the 'herbal antidepressant' St John's wort to be as effective as standard antidepressants such as Prozac.

However, side effects such as dry mouth, dizziness and stomach pains have been widely reported and it interacts strongly with some prescription drugs such as Warfarin and oral contraceptives. And in April, an MHRA investigation into Jia Ji Jian, sometimes marketed as 'herbal Viagra', revealed it contained up to four times the level of pharmaceuticals found in legally prescribed anti-obesity and anti-erectile dysfunction medicinal products, which can cause serious side effects including heart and

THE TELEGRAPH

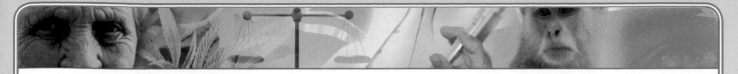

blood pressure problems. As a herbal remedy it should not contain any pharmaceuticals at all.

'Drug interaction is a big area of concern,' says Professor Edzard Ernst, Professor of Complementary Medicine at Exeter University. 'Herbal medicines may have been around for thousands of years, but the new synthetic drugs haven't and how they interact is still uncharted territory.'

The MHRA believes regulating the herbal medicine industry is the best way to limit abuses and ensure consumers are aware of potential dangers. All herbal medicines sold over the counter in the UK should, according to the law, be licensed. The MHRA assesses them on safety, quality and patient information. By 2011 a new scheme, which is currently being rolled out, will be in place.

'Check for products which have the THR (Traditional Herbal Register) or Product Licence (PL) number on the label,' advises Richard Woodfield.

Many herbal practitioners want even further regulation. 'We want to be registered,' says Dee Atkinson, spokesperson for the National Institute of Medical Herbalists and herself a qualified medical herbalist. 'Herbs are not harmless, they are drugs, just as pharmaceuticals are drugs and as such they should be prescribed by a qualified, registered practitioner.

'As a rule of thumb, I'd say that for any conditions or problems you'd normally go to a chemist for, you can visit a shop that sells over-the-counter herbal medicines, but anything beyond that you should be seeing a qualified, and we'd like to see registered, professional. Never order anything off the Internet unless it's from a UK-based, recognised herbal company.'

Richard Woodfield of the MHRA agrees. 'Avoid unlicensed herbal remedies, particularly those sold on the Internet and steer clear of anything claiming to be "100% safe" or "safe because it's natural". Like any other drugs, herbs can have side effects. Look for the THR or PL standard on the label and consult with your doctor if taking any prescription medicine.'

MHRA information line: 020 7084 2000. www.mhra.gov.uk

2 November 2009

© Telegraph Media Group Limited 2010

Call for more research into complementary therapies

New research methods needed to build evidence based on effectiveness of popular complementary therapies.

New research is needed into the clinical and cost effectiveness of the complementary therapies used by millions of Britons every year to improve and manage their health. So says a report by an independent advisory group convened by The King's Fund and chaired by Professor Dame Carol Black published today.

Despite the increasing popularity of treatments like acupuncture, reflexology and osteopathy, the evidence as to whether and how they work is scarce, leaving the practices open to criticism. But lack of agreement on the best methods to test the efficacy and effectiveness of complementary therapies has proved an obstacle to addressing this problem.

This report hopes to establish a consensus on the ways in which research might be conducted that both the conventional and complementary healthcare communities can support.

Explaining the need for different types of research when assessing complementary practice, Professor Dame Carol Black said: 'It has become widely accepted that a stronger evidence base is needed if we are to reach a better understanding of complementary practices and ensure greater confidence in their clinical and cost effectiveness. The challenge is to develop methods of research that allow us to assess the value of an approach that seeks to integrate the physical intervention, the personal context in which it is given, and non-specific effects that together comprise a particular therapy.'

Commenting on the importance of making progress in this area, The King's Fund Chief Executive, Niall Dickson, said: 'Where complementary therapies are offered as part of the NHS it is imperative that those responsible for spending public money base their decisions on sound evidence. We need to understand more about the costs and benefits.

'Doctors and patients need robust evidence to make informed decisions – more research will play a vital role in showing what works and what does not, what is cost effective and what is not.'

The report is the result of debate between experts in the fields of medical research, funding and practice, and was conducted over the course of more than two years.

10 August 2009

⇨ The above information is reprinted with kind permission from The King's Fund. Visit www.kingsfund.org.uk for more information.

© The King's Fund

THE TELEGRAPH / THE KING'S FUND

Complementary medicine: health risk or the real heal?

A controversial book questions the value of complementary medicine, says Jane Alexander.

Do you receive reiki or put your feet in the hands of a reflexologist? Have you ever tried crystal therapy? Does an acupuncturist give you a needle? In short, are you one of the estimated 5.75 million people in Britain who visit a complementary health practitioner?

If so, according to Professor Edzard Ernst and Simon Singh, authors of *Trick or Treatment*, you're not only potentially wasting your money, you could be putting your health at risk.

'Millions of patients are wasting their money and risking their health by turning towards a snake-oil industry,' they say.

Unsurprisingly, practitioners of complementary medicine have been less than ecstatic about the authors' stance.

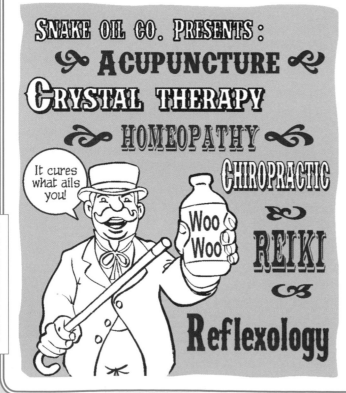

The British Chiropractic Association (BCA) accused Singh of libel over an article he wrote in the *Guardian*.

The BCA claimed he was, in effect, accusing chiropractors of knowingly supporting bogus treatments. The Court of Appeal has ruled that Singh can use the 'defence of fair comment' in the ongoing dispute.

While Singh is a science writer and documentary maker, Ernst is Professor of Complementary Medicine at Exeter University. Qualified as a conventional doctor, he consequently trained in homeopathy and practised this and other therapies.

However, as he looked at the research, he became 'increasingly disillusioned'.

His main complaint is that, according to his reviews of the available research, it simply doesn't work. If people get better, they do so because of the placebo effect or by sheer coincidence.

Homeopathy, Ernst says, 'makes no scientific sense'. He also claims it can be dangerous because it can prevent patients seeking medical attention for serious ailments.

Acupuncture, he continues, is also fundamentally unproven by clinical trials. In addition, if wrongly performed, Ernst says it can cause infection and that needles might even puncture a nerve or an organ.

Chiropractic also comes in for a panning (you can understand why they took umbrage). Ernst expresses concern if patients are being X-rayed unnecessarily, and adds: 'patients can also suffer dislocations and fractures'. Herbs, he concedes, can have physiological effects and a few, such as St John's wort, Devil's Claw, Echinacea, garlic, ginkgo and horse chestnut, do respond well in trials.

However, he points out that herbal treatments have side-effects and that some herbs interact badly with conventional medicine.

The 50 per cent of doctors who refer patients to therapists

THE TELEGRAPH

of unproven treatments receive a lambasting, with Ernst suggesting that they are either ignorant, lazy or desperate.

Prince Charles, a long-term advocate of complementary health, also gets an earful. 'The Prince of Wales ought to start listening to scientists, rather than allowing himself to be guided by his own prejudices.' Ouch.

It's based on science, so surely Ernst must be right? Well, not everyone agrees that it's that simple. Professor George Lewith is Professor of Health Research at the University of Southampton – hence in the same business as Ernst.

While Lewith firmly believes that complementary medicine 'should be trialled and tested', he expresses concern about the scientific basis of *Trick or Treatment*.

'Synthesising one or two rather inadequate trials and coming to a negative conclusion is a very limited and often inaccurate way to look at clinical evidence,' Lewith says. 'The honest answer when we have inadequate evidence is that we don't know. Ernst routinely spins "don't know" into "doesn't work" by implication and this theme tends to run through *Trick or Treatment*.'

So are these therapies safe after all? 'If we applied the same scientific rules used in *Trick or Treatment* to surgical intervention, we would probably never agree to let a dentist or indeed any surgeon ever approach us,' Lewith says with a shrug.

'All medicine needs to be aware that it should operate safely and honestly, but Ernst and Singh seem to be waging some sort of religious war against complementary medicine.'

The book does seem curiously slanted. Ernst mentions in passing that some forms of complementary health do produce measurable results – osteopathy, massage therapies, yoga and autogenic therapy fare reasonably well, for example.

Yet the praise is faint.

I, for one, would have felt more convinced by the negative commentary if there had been more emphasis on the parts of complementary health that do seem to stand up to rigorous testing.

There was also little acknowledgement of why some patients seek natural therapies in the first place.

While pharmaceutical drugs are extensively tested in the manner Ernst approves, they are scarcely devoid of side-effects. Also, many people seek help for issues that conventional medicine finds difficult to treat.

Research shows that the most common ailments seen by complementary practitioners are musculoskeletal problems, stress, anxiety and depression. Interestingly, these are all conditions that respond well to the therapies which were given grudging applause in *Trick or Treatment*.

The bottom line? It seems the jury is still out.

Trick or Treatment? Alternative Medicine on Trial by Simon Singh and Edzard Ernst is published by Corgi (£7.99)

Professor Ernst likes:

⇨ Autogenic training – 'An economical self-help approach.'

⇨ Massage – 'Improves well-being in most patients.'

⇨ Meditation – 'Can be useful for many people.'

⇨ Osteopathy – 'The osteopathic approach is effective for back pain.'

⇨ Leech therapy – 'Some evidence shows this treatment reduces the pain of osteoarthritis.'

Professor Ernst dislikes:

⇨ Bach Flower remedies – 'Flower remedies are a waste of money.'

⇨ Colonic irrigation – 'Unpleasant, ineffective.'

⇨ Crystal therapy – 'Based on irrational mystical concepts.'

⇨ Reflexology – 'Offers nothing more than could be achieved by a simple, relaxing foot massage.'

⇨ Reiki – 'Has no basis in science.'

Can meditation help depression?

⇨ The effectiveness of meditation as a treatment for depression is supported by research. A study at the University of California, Los Angeles, of Transcendental Meditation (TM) shows that this form of meditation can reduce the symptoms of depression by 50 per cent over a 12-month period.

⇨ It isn't cheap to learn (between £390 and £590) and has cultish associations.

⇨ The UCLA study didn't compare TM with other forms of meditation but you can achieve equally impressive benefits with less cost.

⇨ Try mindfulness, a technique developed at the University of Massachusetts Medical School. The Mental Health Foundation would like to see courses in this effective self-help treatment run by the NHS.

⇨ Meanwhile you can learn it from *Wherever You Go, There You Are* by Jon Kabat-Zinn (Piatkus) £12.99.

⇨ For more about TM, call 01695 51213; www.t-m.org. uk. For more about mindfulness, see www.bemindful. co.uk

16 April 2010

© Telegraph Media Group Limited 2010

THE TELEGRAPH

BMA votes against homeopathy funding

The British Medical Association (BMA) has called for homeopathic remedies to be banned on the NHS and removed from pharmacies where they are for sale as medicines.

Medics at a BMA conference voted overwhelmingly in favour of banning homeopathic remedies being funded by the NHS and withdrawing backing for the UK's four homeopathic hospitals. They added that NHS doctors should not be given homeopathy training and remedies should be taken off shelves 'labelled medicines' and put on shelves 'labelled placebos'.

Homeopathic treatments have been funded by the NHS since it was formed in 1948 and are different to herbal medicine as they are based around substances being diluted many times, something the conference claimed has been proven not to work.

MPs said back in February that the NHS should withdraw funding on homeopathic treatments as there is no substantial evidence to show that they work any better than a placebo – the same as taking a sugar or dummy pill and believing it works. They also said the Medicines and Healthcare products Regulatory Agency (MHRA) should not allow homeopathic medicines to carry medical claims on their labels.

In the UK, London, Bristol, Liverpool and Glasgow all house homeopathic hospitals. Estimates on how much the NHS spends on homeopathy vary, with the Society of Homeopaths putting the figure at £4 million a year including the cost of running hospitals.

30 June 2010

⇨ The above information is reprinted with kind permission from *Nursing Times*. Visit their website at www.nursingtimes.net for more information on this and other related topics.

© Nursing Times

EU to fund complementary medicine research

The Prince's Foundation for Integrated Health welcomes news that the EU is to put €1.5 million into complementary medicine research over the next three years.

Called CAMbrella, the plan is to create a network of European research institutes that will focus on patients' needs, the role of complementary and alternative medicine (CAM) in healthcare systems, legal regulation, research methodology and terminology.

Professor George Lewith, who heads the CAM research unit at Southampton University, is one of the project's co-ordinators and a Foundation Fellow. He said:

'More than 100 million people in Europe and the UK are regular users of complementary and alternative medicine.

'Yet compared with conventional medicine, there is a lack of research, very little funding and not enough scientific co-operation.

'That cannot be good for patients' safety.'

Lead co-ordinator Dr. Wolfgang Weidenhammer, Centre of Naturheilkunde, Technische Universität, Munich, Germany, said:

'We will develop a comprehensive understanding of the current status of CAM in Europe, which will serve as a starting point for future healthcare delivery and research.'

The research group consists of 16 scientific partner organisations from 12 European countries. The UK is represented by Southampton University Medical School. The project is supported by an Advisory Board, which includes members of the relevant stakeholder organisations such as patient and practitioner organisations, providers and consumers.

January 2010

⇨ The above information is reprinted with kind permission from the Prince's Fund for Integrated Health. Visit www.fih.org.uk for more information.

© Prince's Fund for Integrated Health

NURSING TIMES / PRINCE'S FUND FOR INTEGRATED HEALTH

Supporters of homeopathy outraged at medical union's attacks

Information from the British Homeopathic Association.

British supporters of homeopathy, including GPs, medical experts, MPs and patients, are disappointed by motions carried against homeopathy at today's conference of the British Medical Association in Brighton.

Many supporters of homeopathy gathered in front of the Brighton Centre with banners and placards to let doctors know that they value NHS homeopathy, which has improved their health, and they should consider patients when voting today.

The motions specifically demand that NHS funding for homeopathic remedies and homeopathic hospitals is banned and that there should be no homeopathic training posts available in NHS hospitals.

Homeopathy, which has been available on the NHS since the formation of the health service in 1948, is an extremely small part of the NHS budget

Dr Sara Eames, President of the Faculty of Homeopathy, the organisation which represents doctors that practise homeopathy, stated: 'I am shocked and disappointed that my profession's trade union should pass these motions without consulting doctors who practise homeopathy or allowing them to participate in the debate. There is a growing evidence base for homeopathy with far more positive than negative trials, increasing laboratory evidence and most importantly of all the large numbers of patients who have been helped by homeopathy when all other treatments have failed. What will happen to these patients now? Is patient choice to become the domain of the wealthy?'

Homeopathy, which has been available on the NHS since the formation of the health service in 1948, is an extremely small part of the NHS budget, with homeopathic medicines making up 0.001% of the NHS drugs budget. Hundreds of doctors throughout the UK practise homeopathy, providing approximately 60,000 patients with homeopathic care through the NHS. Without access to NHS homeopathy these patients would be referred to more expensive specialists and be prescribed more costly conventional medicine.

Television presenter and former tennis star Annabel Croft said: 'I'm shocked to hear that treatments that benefit tens of thousands of people across the UK are under threat, as homeopathy has been proven to work for a wide range of ailments. The option to choose a more holistic approach to medicine should not be taken away from millions of potential patients who could benefit.'

'While this country grapples with serious challenges in funding the NHS amounting to billions of pounds, the BMA is choosing to launch an unfair attack on a field of treatment that helps thousands of people in a very cost-effective way,' said Cristal Sumner, Chief Executive of the British Homeopathic Association. 'It saddens me that the BMA with no consultation and only ten minutes, debating time decided to pass motions that could have a hugely detrimental effect on the millions of patients and thousands of doctors that use homeopathy. I hope the government has more sense and concern for patients than to endorse these recommendations.'

29 June 2010

⇨ The above information is reprinted with kind permission from the British Homeopathic Association. Visit www.britishhomeopathic.org for more information.

© British Homeopathic Association

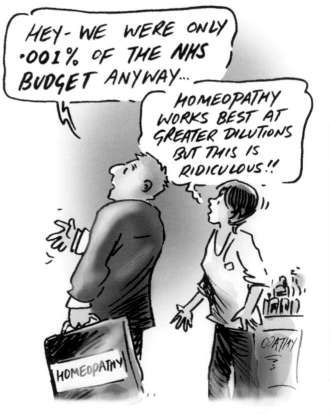

BRITISH HOMEOPATHIC ASSOCIATION

An overview of NHS homeopathy

Information from the British Homeopathic Association.

NHS homeopathic hospitals

As well as around 400 GPs who integrate homeopathy into their practice in the UK, there are four NHS homeopathic hospitals – Bristol, Liverpool, London and Glasgow. All have been part of the NHS since it was founded in 1948, though many of them have existed for over 100 years. These are consultant-led services staffed by fully qualified doctors, nurses and other healthcare professionals who have additional training in homeopathy and other complementary therapies such as acupuncture. Patients are referred, as is usual in the NHS, by their GP or specialist.

The homeopathic hospitals are a unique asset to the NHS, for several reasons:

⇨ They offer patients genuine choice of treatment by providing evidence-based, highly professional complementary medicine. Most patients are unable to afford private treatment.

⇨ Although small they are highly innovative: for instance acupuncture for pain and complementary cancer care, both now widely available in the NHS, were pioneered by the homeopathic hospitals.

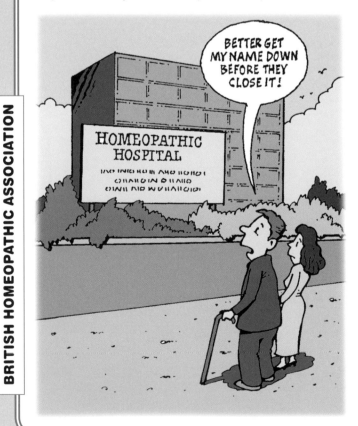

⇨ They have made important research contributions, for instance researching 'effectiveness gaps' – conditions for which GPs lack effective treatments, and the outcome and cost-effectiveness of complementary medicine.

The hospitals help many patients who have been failed by other parts of the NHS – including those with complex chronic problems and for whom conventional medicine has proved ineffective or associated with serious side-effects. The treatments offered by the homeopathic hospitals are complementary to, and integrated with, conventional treatment. Treatment is provided by qualified healthcare professionals working within the NHS.

Hospitals at risk

In the past the Government has re-affirmed its commitment to homeopathy in the NHS – a commitment originally made by Aneurin Bevan, the architect of the health service. Speaking on 7 April 1977, Eric Deakins (Under Secretary of State for Health) said: 'Homeopathic treatment should be available under the NHS as long as there are practitioners who are willing to provide it and patients wishing to receive it.' (*Hansard* 1977)

As well as around 400 GPs who integrate homeopathy into their practice in the UK, there are four NHS homeopathic hospitals – Bristol, Liverpool, London and Glasgow

However, local NHS commissioning and the financial crisis currently affecting the NHS have placed these unique national assets at risk. Decisions that affect patients' ability to choose their treatment are being made to satisfy short-term financial needs by NHS commissioners who have little understanding of the value the homeopathic hospitals provide.

Negative media coverage

There is concern that NHS commissioners have been encouraged to make cuts by a series of high-profile hostile leaks to the media. These include a leak of a draft of the Smallwood Report, by the economist Christopher Smallwood, highlighting the potential of complementary therapies to provide cost-effective NHS treatment options, which was commissioned by the Prince's Foundation for Integrated Health (front page of the *Times,* 25 August 2005).

BRITISH HOMEOPATHIC ASSOCIATION

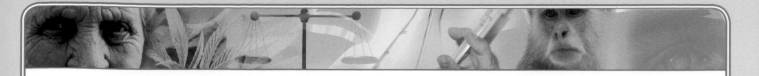

There was also a letter attacking complementary medicine, sent to chief executives of all Primary Care Trusts and leaked, again on the front page of the *Times*, on 23 May 2006, which used the NHS logo without permission from the Department of Health (DH). DH later called the use of the logo 'inappropriate'. This was followed by an 'anniversary' letter on 23 May 2007 to the same PCTs which was also widely reported.

The long-term impact could be an irreversible loss of patient choice which will leave many patients stranded – particularly those for whom conventional medicine has failed.

Fragmented policy

The amounts of money involved are tiny. In Tunbridge Wells, West Kent Primary Care Trust cancelled its £196,000 a year contract with the homeopathic hospital there, despite a vigorous local campaign and public consultation results which favoured keeping homeopathy funding. This contract accounted for 50% of the patients seen at Tunbridge Wells and its loss meant that the service was no longer viable – the hospital closed in March 2009.

Other homeopathic hospitals are facing similar decisions by PCTs seeking to reduce costs. This is being done without considering the additional resources that will be consumed elsewhere in the NHS as a consequence of patients being refused treatment at the homeopathic hospitals. Because of the fragmented nature of NHS commissioning arrangements, no one body has oversight of this, or of the potential consequence of the irreversible loss of these small, unique units which punch far above their weight in terms of patient care, innovation and research.

Comparing numbers

NHS spending on homeopathy is very small. The service lost at Tunbridge Wells equates to around 0.0002% of the NHS's total budget.

⇨ Total NHS budget: £100 billion.

⇨ Annual spend on inpatients with adverse reactions to drugs: £466 million.

⇨ Annual spend on management consultants: £300 million.

⇨ Annual spend on homeopathy: £4 million.

⇨ Cost of Tunbridge Wells Homeopathic Hospital contract with PCT: £196,000.

The contracts the homeopathic hospitals have with Primary Care Trusts are a minuscule proportion of the NHS budget – and yet make such a big difference to patients. Outcome studies from the hospitals consistently show that well over two-thirds of patients feel better after treatment.

⇨ The above information is reprinted with kind permission from the British Homeopathic Association. Visit www.britishhomeopathic.org for more information on this and other related topics.

© British Homeopathic Association

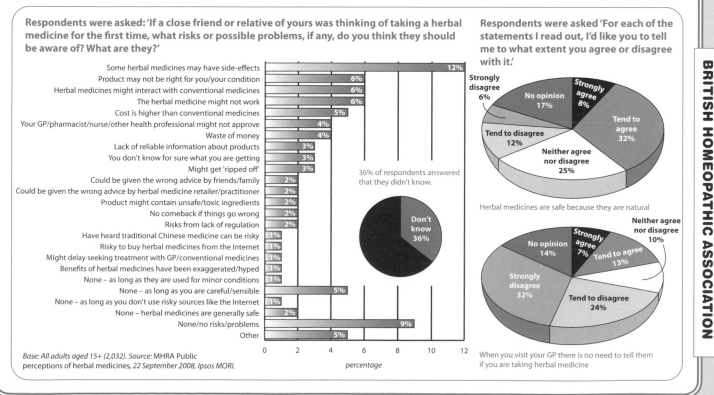

Respondents were asked: 'If a close friend or relative of yours was thinking of taking a herbal medicine for the first time, what risks or possible problems, if any, do you think they should be aware of? What are they?'

	percentage
Some herbal medicines may have side-effects	12%
Product may not be right for you/your condition	6%
Herbal medicines might interact with conventional medicines	6%
The herbal medicine might not work	6%
Cost is higher than conventional medicines	5%
Your GP/pharmacist/nurse/other health professional might not approve	4%
Waste of money	4%
Lack of reliable information about products	3%
You don't know for sure what you are getting	3%
Might get 'ripped off'	3%
Could be given the wrong advice by friends/family	2%
Could be given the wrong advice by herbal medicine retailer/practitioner	2%
Product might contain unsafe/toxic ingredients	2%
No comeback if things go wrong	2%
Risks from lack of regulation	2%
Have heard traditional Chinese medicine can be risky	1%
Risky to buy herbal medicines from the Internet	1%
Might delay seeking treatment with GP/conventional medicines	1%
Benefits of herbal medicines have been exaggerated/hyped	1%
None – as long as they are used for minor conditions	1%
None – as long as you are careful/sensible	5%
None – as long as you don't use risky sources like the Internet	1%
None – herbal medicines are generally safe	2%
None/no risks/problems	9%
Other	5%

36% of respondents answered that they didn't know.

Don't know 36%

Base: All adults aged 15+ (2,032). Source: MHRA Public perceptions of herbal medicines, 22 September 2008, Ipsos MORI.

Respondents were asked 'For each of the statements I read out, I'd like you to tell me to what extent you agree or disagree with it.'

Strongly disagree 6%
No opinion 17%
Strongly agree 8%
Tend to agree 32%
Tend to disagree 12%
Neither agree nor disagree 25%

Herbal medicines are safe because they are natural

No opinion 14%
Strongly agree 7%
Neither agree nor disagree 10%
Tend to agree 13%
Strongly disagree 32%
Tend to disagree 24%

When you visit your GP there is no need to tell them if you are taking herbal medicine

BRITISH HOMEOPATHIC ASSOCIATION

Ban homeopathy on NHS, say MPs

Homeopathy should no longer be available on the NHS, according to MPs on the Commons Science and Technology Committee.

In a report published today, the cross-party committee says by funding homeopathic treatments, the Government is giving the impression that they work.

'By providing homeopathy on the NHS and allowing MHRA (Medicines and Healthcare products Regulatory Agency) licensing of products which subsequently appear on pharmacy shelves, the Government runs the risk of endorsing homeopathy as an efficacious system of medicine.

'To maintain patient trust, choice and safety, the Government should not endorse the use of placebo treatments, including homeopathy. Homeopathy should not be funded on the NHS and the MHRA should stop licensing homeopathic products.'

The Health Department told the committee that it 'does not maintain a position' on any complementary or alternative treatment, including homeopathy. Decisions are left to the NHS, with primary care trusts given the freedom to fund homeopathy if they choose.

'To maintain patient trust, choice and safety, the Government should not endorse the use of placebo treatments, including homeopathy'

Costs unclear

Homeopathy has been available on the NHS since it was formed in 1948, but exactly what it is costing the taxpayer is not clear. The Health Minister Mike O'Brien told the committee: 'In terms of drugs, it is £152,000 a year, which comes from a budget of £11bn. It is approximately 0.001 per cent, we calculated, of the drugs budget. In terms of overall funding, it is very difficult to know.

'We have done some work to see if we can find out what it is. We have four hospitals – one in Glasgow, three in England – which provide homeopathic assistance to people and we do provide some NHS funding for those, so it would run into several million on that basis.'

Last year, the *Guardian* newspaper reported that the NHS spent £12m on homeopathy from 2005-08. The Society of Homeopaths estimates that £4m is spent annually. But the committee says: 'It appears that these figures do not include maintenance and running costs of the homeopathic hospitals or the £20m spent on refurbishing the Royal London Homeopathic Hospital between 2002 and 2005.'

The other homeopathic hospitals in Britain are in Bristol and Liverpool.

NHS has funded homeopathy since 1948

The committee's report says: 'The NHS funds homeopathy and has done so since 1948. We were disappointed that, in light of its view on evidence for homeopathy, the Government has no appetite to review its policies in favour of an evidence-based approach.

'The Government was reluctant to address the issues of informed patient choice or the appropriateness and ethics of prescribing placebos to patients. We would expect the Government to have a view on the efficacy of homeopathy so as to inform its policy on the NHS funding and provision of homeopathy.'

Reviews suggest that homeopathic products are no better than placebos, say the MPs.

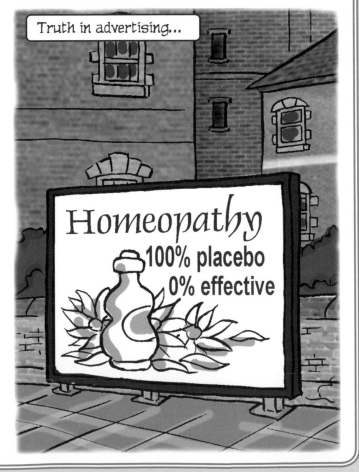

Truth in advertising...

Homeopathy
100% placebo
0% effective

CHANNEL 4

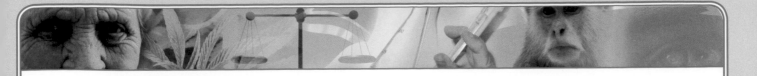

'We regret that advocates of homeopathy, including in their submissions to our inquiry, choose to rely on, and promulgate, selective approaches to the treatment of the evidence base as this risks confusing or misleading the public, the media and policy-makers.

'There has been enough testing of homeopathy and plenty of evidence showing that it is not efficacious. Competition for research funding is fierce and we cannot see how further research on the efficacy of homeopathy is justified in the face of competing priorities.

'We do not doubt that homeopathy makes some patients feel better. However, patient satisfaction can occur through a placebo effect alone and therefore does not prove the efficacy of homeopathic interventions.

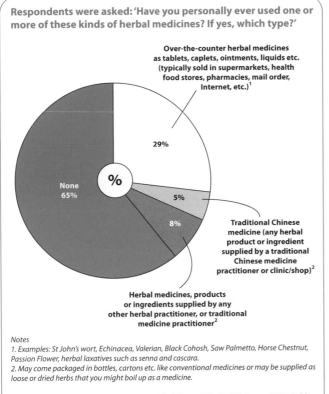

Respondents were asked: 'Have you personally ever used one or more of these kinds of herbal medicines? If yes, which type?'

Over-the-counter herbal medicines as tablets, caplets, ointments, liquids etc. (typically sold in supermarkets, health food stores, pharmacies, mail order, Internet, etc.)[1]

29%

None 65%

%

5%

8%

Traditional Chinese medicine (any herbal product or ingredient supplied by a traditional Chinese medicine practitioner or clinic/shop)[2]

Herbal medicines, products or ingredients supplied by any other herbal practitioner, or traditional medicine practitioner[2]

Notes
1. Examples: St John's wort, Echinacea, Valerian, Black Cohosh, Saw Palmetto, Horse Chestnut, Passion Flower, herbal laxatives such as senna and cascara.
2. May come packaged in bottles, cartons etc. like conventional medicines or may be supplied as loose or dried herbs that you might boil up as a medicine.

Base: All adults aged 15+ (2,032). Source: MHRA Public perceptions of herbal medicines, 22 September 2008, Ipsos MORI.

'For patient choice to be real choice, patients must be adequately informed to understand the implications of treatments. For homeopathy this would certainly require an explanation that homeopathy is a placebo. When this is not done, patient choice is meaningless.'

Stop referring to homeopaths

'By funding homeopathy, the NHS is endorsing it.

'Since the NHS Constitution explicitly gives people the right to expect that decisions on the funding of drugs and treatments are made "following a proper consideration of the evidence", patients may reasonably form the view that homeopathy is an evidence-based treatment.

'The Government should stop allowing the funding of homeopathy on the NHS. We conclude that placebos should not be routinely prescribed on the NHS. The funding of homeopathic hospitals – hospitals that specialise in the administration of placebos – should not continue, and NHS doctors should not refer patients to homeopaths.

'We consider that the way to deal with the sale of homeopathic products is to remove any medical claim and any implied endorsement of efficacy by the MHRA – other than where its evidential standards used to assess conventional medicines have been met – and for the labelling to make it explicit that there is no scientific evidence.'

Channel 4 News science correspondent Tom Clarke writes:

What's really interesting about the committee's finding is that they haven't found that homeopathy is totally ineffective. They've found that homeopathy does help some people because it's a very powerful placebo.

People receiving homeopathic treatment can think they're getting better.

Now, defenders of the treatment will dispute that. But moderates would say well, in that case, why not support the continued use of homeopathy in the NHS? It doesn't cost much and it makes people feel better.

And that's where the committee strongly disagree. They say the NHS should base its policies on good scientific evidence – and for homeopathy there is none.

They also concluded that there was nothing specifically directly harmful with homeopathic treatments because they are, after all, only water.

But they did find there was a potential for institutional harm, given that acceptance of homeopathy could be 'toxic to a system' that is meant to ensure that medicines are not just safe but effective.

Many supporters of homeopathic remedies see this as motivated by a group of fundamentalist scientists. They say there is still need for more research on the benefits of homeopathy and questions like 'water memory' that underpin it.

However, the committee argues that asking bodies like NICE to look into homeopathy would be a further waste of money, given the lack of any existing scientific evidence.

22 February 2010

⇨ The above information is reprinted with kind permission from Channel 4. Visit www.channel4.com for more information.

© *Channel 4*

CHANNEL 4

Homeopathy works and is an important part of the NHS

Information from the British Homeopathic Association.

Homeopathy is more than a placebo and rightfully belongs in the NHS where patients can best benefit from doctors integrating it into care.

The British Homeopathic Association is astonished by the recommendations in the Science and Technology Committee report, which fails to acknowledge the fact that research evidence for homeopathy does exist, and which dismisses patient outcomes as placebo effect.

The majority of patients presenting at the NHS homeopathic hospitals have serious and chronic conditions that have often not been helped through conventional methods. These patients are not – as the committee would like to purport – presenting with minor complaints whose improvement is easily explained away by a placebo response.

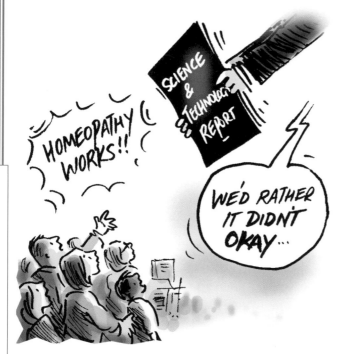

The review by the committee was very narrow and cursory. The committee did not entertain evidence of effectiveness, which is actually what patients care most about. Even more troubling, the committee's report makes recommendations to government in isolation of context and apparently without concern about its impact on patients and the NHS. If homeopathic patients are pushed to other, more expensive, services, how will it help the NHS funding crisis? What about patients who have found nothing but homeopathy has helped them?

Homeopathy has been part of the NHS since its inception and has helped hundreds of thousands of people. In the NHS, homeopathy is provided by Faculty of Homeopathy doctors, which is the best and safest way to access such care.

Chief Executive Cristal Sumner states: 'It does seem an irresponsible way of decision-making for a committee of four voting members to draw conclusions that impact the health and welfare of thousands of patients from just four and a half hours of verbal testimony on three distinct topics and from a number of written submissions that were each limited to just 3,000 words.'

As the Health Minister, Mike O'Brien, said, it would be illiberal to cut funding. We at the BHA know patients benefit from homeopathy, we hear their stories daily, and emphatically believe patients should retain their right to access homeopathy on the NHS.

British Homeopathic Association

The British Homeopathic Association (BHA) is a registered charity, which aims to ensure high-quality homeopathy is an integral part of general and specialist healthcare. The BHA works towards this goal by providing information to the public, promoting access to treatment and supporting the homeopathic education of healthcare professionals and research. www.britishhomeopathic. org

The Faculty of Homeopathy

The Faculty of Homeopathy, incorporated by Act of Parliament in 1950, accredits and sets standards for doctors, vets, nurses, midwives, dentists, pharmacists, podiatrists and other healthcare professionals who use homeopathic medicine. The Faculty promotes an integrated approach to care across all medical fields, where homeopathy is used to complement conventional medicine. www.facultyofhomeopathy.org

22 February 2010

⇨ The above information is reprinted with kind permission from the British Homeopathic Association. Visit www.britishhomeopathic.org for more information.

© British Homeopathic Association

BRITISH HOMEOPATHIC ASSOCIATION

Government urged to embrace integrated healthcare

Conservative MP David Tredinnick writes for ePolitix.com ahead of his adjournment debate on integrated healthcare.

For the first time in a general election, integrated healthcare and more specifically homeopathic medical treatments were issues. The arch critic of homeopathy, Evan Harris (Oxford and Abingdon), lost his seat by 176 votes. Not only had he angered many voters by his illiberal, and some say irrational, views, but a number of therapists actively campaigned against him – and with spectacular results.

In my own constituency the Science Party candidate who campaigned against my support for integrated health care, complementary medicine and, yes, homeopathy, lost his deposit.

Surveys show that support for a healthcare model that allows doctors to refer to other therapists such as herbalists, acupuncturists, homeopaths and aromatherapists is increasing. The new coalition Government seeking to both give more say to doctors and more choice to patients should embrace integrated healthcare as its model.

> **Surveys show that support for a healthcare model that allows doctors to refer to other therapists such as herbalists, acupuncturists, homeopaths and aromatherapists is increasing**

The proposed Independent NHS Board, there to allocate resources and provide commissioning guidance, should offer guidance on integrated healthcare, and to GPs who will be allowed to commission services on behalf of patients – the better the regulation the more likely GPs are to refer.

The new Government must attend to the unfinished business of the old, and in particular the regulation of herbal medicine and acupuncturists which has been the subject of several enquiries in recent years. The last Government's proposal to regulate practitioners through the Complementary and Natural Healthcare Council (CNHC) instead of the Health Professionals Council (HPC) was a mistake. The bodies representing the Chinese medical community, such as the Association of Traditional Chinese Medicine (ATCM) want the higher standards of the HPC.

> **In France homeopathy is taught in seven medical schools and practised by 25,000 doctors**

The homeopathic practitioners have different issues. The much criticised Science and Technology Select Committee report *Evidence Check 2: Homeopathy* (HC45:Feb 2010) was promoted by defeated MP Evan Harris. The criticism set out in EDM 908, signed by 70 Members, centred on the report's failure to take evidence from practitioners, that it ignored successful randomised controlled trials, and that it took no account at all of the widespread and increasing use of homeopathy in Europe and elsewhere. For example, in France homeopathy is taught in seven medical schools and practised by 25,000 doctors. In India there are 180 colleges teaching homeopathy and over 300,000 practitioners.

Other issues to be considered include food supplements and other related EC legislation, the need to facilitate the statutory or voluntary regulations of therapies including aromatherapy, hypnotherapy and reiki.

Finally, the last Conservative Government took the first steps towards integrated healthcare when in 1990 the then Parliamentary Under Secretary of State For Health, Stephen Dorrell (Charnwood), allowed doctors to refer to complementary therapists provided they accepted clinical responsibility. This Government can complete the process by putting in place sound regulations, by providing good advice and direction. And by ensuring that cost-effective and medically effective acupuncture, herbal medicine, homeopathy and other therapies form part of a truly integrated health service.

2 June 2010

⇨ The above information is reprinted with kind permission from ePolitix. Visit www.epolitix.com for more information.

© ePolitix

EPOLITIX

Homeopathy remains on NHS

Information from the NHS Knowledge Service – 'Behind the Headlines'.

'Homeopathy will continue to be available on the NHS despite an influential health committee condemning it as medically unproven,' reported the *Daily Telegraph*.

The newspaper, together with several other media outlets, was reporting the Department of Health's response to a report by the House of Commons cross-party Select Committee on Science and Technology, published in February.

That committee had said homeopathic medicine should no longer be funded on the NHS and called for a ban on the medicines carrying medical claims on their labels.

It found no evidence the medicines are any more effective than a placebo (the same as taking a sugar pill and believing it works). The British Medical Association agreed, with a leading member recently describing homeopathy as 'witchcraft'.

> **'We believe in patients being able to make informed choices about their treatments, and in a clinician being able to prescribe the treatment they feel most appropriate'**

The Department of Health based its decision to continue funding homeopathy on 'choice', not efficacy, reported the newspapers.

'We believe in patients being able to make informed choices about their treatments, and in a clinician being able to prescribe the treatment they feel most appropriate in particular circumstances,' said a spokesman.

'Our continued position on the use of homeopathy within the NHS is that the local NHS and clinicians, rather than Whitehall, are best placed to make decisions on what treatment is appropriate for their patients.'

What is homeopathy?

Homeopathy is a type of complementary and alternative medicine (CAM). CAMs are treatments that are not part of conventional Western medicine. Like most CAMs, homeopathy's use and efficacy (how well it works in placebo-controlled trials) are controversial, and most mainstream scientists reject it as a concept and consider that it only works because of the placebo effect.

What's the idea behind it?

Homeopaths believe that homeopathy can help with any condition that the body has the potential to repair itself. The practice has two essential principles:

⇨ That a substance that can cause symptoms of illness will cure those same symptoms if given in extremely small doses. For example, a very small amount of caffeine might be used to treat insomnia.

⇨ The more you dilute a substance, the more you increase its power to treat symptoms that it would otherwise cause. The dilution of the substance must be performed in a very specific way, with an increasing number of dilutions resulting in the solution becoming more potent.

To what extent are the substances diluted?

Ben Goldacre, the author of *Bad Science*, has described the process:

'The typical dilution is called "30C": this means that the original substance has been diluted by 1 drop in 100, 30 times. On the Society of Homeopaths site, in their 'What is homeopathy?' section, they say that "30C contains less than 1 part per million of the original substance."

'This is an understatement: a 30C homeopathic preparation is a dilution of 1 in 100^{30}, or rather 1 in 10^{60}, which means a 1 followed by 60 zeroes, or – let's be absolutely clear – a dilution of 1 in 1,000,000,000, 000,000,000,000,000,000,000,000,000, 000,000,000, 000,000,000,000,000.

'To phrase that in the Society of Homeopaths' terms, we should say: "30C contains less than one part per million million million million million million million million million million of the original substance."

'At a homeopathic dilution of 100C, which they sell routinely, and which homeopaths claim is even more powerful than 30C, the treating substance is diluted by more than the total number of atoms in the universe. Homeopathy was invented before we knew what atoms were, or how many there are, or how big they are. It has not changed its belief system in light of this information.'

Why do people accuse homeopaths of witchcraft?

The phrase is pejorative. Some people use it because

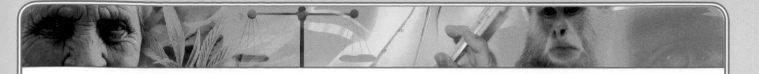

the process of creating homeopathic medicines involves unusual traditions, such as knocking the solution against a leather and horsehair surface during the dilution process.

What's the major criticism of homeopathy?

The key criticism is that there is no reliable scientific evidence to suggest it is any more effective than a placebo. Normally, drugs that are no more effective than a placebo are judged ineffective and not given a licence or funded by the NHS. Prescribing placebo treatments, critics say, damages the trust that exists between doctors and their patients.

Critics of homeopathy say the reason the medicines are ineffective is because in homeopathic remedies the original substance is diluted to such an extent that no molecules of the substance remain in the remedy.

Homeopaths have argued that the critics are missing the point of the dilution process. The homeopaths claim it is not necessary for any of the original substance to remain as the dilution process somehow imprints a 'memory' of the substance into the water.

What did the Select Committee on Science and Technology conclude?

The Select Committee on Science and Technology concluded that:

⇨ There is no evidence that homeopathy works beyond the placebo effect, which is a position that the Government agrees with.

⇨ By providing homeopathy on the NHS, the Government runs the risk of appearing to endorse it as a working system of medicine. There is also the danger that when doctors prescribe placebos, they risk damaging the trust that exists between them and their patients.

⇨ Given that the existing scientific literature shows no good evidence of efficacy, further clinical trials of homeopathy are not justified.

What was the Government's response?

The Government has decided to continue to allow homeopathic hospitals and treatments to be received on the NHS, where local doctors recommend them.

It agrees that the efficacy of a treatment is important, but said there are many considerations when making policy decisions, and that patient choice is an important factor to consider.

'We believe that providing appropriate information for commissioners, clinicians and the public, and ensuring a strong ethical code for clinicians, remain the most effective ways to ensure quality outcomes, patient satisfaction and the appropriate use of NHS funding.'

The Government also said that it noted the Committee's view that allowing for the provision of homeopathy may risk seeming to endorse it, and that it would keep the position under review.

What does the Government Chief Scientific Adviser say?

The Government Chief Scientific Adviser has expressed his concern that the public may assume that NHS homeopathic treatments are 'efficacious', whereas the principal reason for their availability is to provide patient choice.

Homeopaths believe that homeopathy can help with any condition that the body has the potential to repair itself

To enable the public to make informed choices, he will work with the Department of Health to ensure that the public has access to clear information on the evidence for homeopathy.

His position, as stated in the Government response, remains that 'the evidence of efficacy and the scientific basis of homeopathy is highly questionable'.

What do homeopaths say?

On their website, the British Homeopathic Association say: 'Today's response by Government to the Science and Technology Committee report *Evidence Check 2: Homeopathy* reaffirms homeopathy belongs in the NHS where patients can best benefit from doctors integrating it into healthcare.'

How much does homeopathy cost the NHS each year?

Exact figures for the cost of homeopathy are not collected. However, there are currently four homeopathic hospitals in England, and in the region of 25,000 homeopathic items are prescribed each year. Total costs are thought to be in the region of £3-4 million a year.

4 August 2010

⇨ Reproduced by kind permission of the Department of Health.

© Crown copyright – nhs.uk 2010

NHS

Government ignored our advice on homeopathic remedies, say experts

Treatments still funded on NHS despite lack of proof that they work.

By Steve Connor, Science Editor

The coalition Government ignored scientific advice on the questionable nature of homeopathy by continuing to allow the NHS to fund homeopathic treatment despite there being next to no evidence that it works, leading scientists have told *The Independent*.

Last week, health ministers refused calls from the House of Commons science and technology committee to stop the NHS funding homeopathic treatment on the grounds that such a ban would limit patient choice and contradict the Government's stated aim of devolving more power to the Primary Care Trusts (PCTs) of the NHS.

However, the Government's own chief scientific adviser, Sir John Beddington, said that he had spoken informally to coalition ministers about his grave concerns over homeopathy and the Department of Health's policy of allowing it to be prescribed under the NHS.

'I remain of the view that the evidence of efficacy and the scientific evidence base of homeopathy is highly questionable. It is vitally important that the public can make informed choices on their use of homeopathy, so the evidence base must be freely available in an easily-accessible format,' Sir John said.

The Government does not know how many PCTs prescribe homeopathic treatment or how much it costs but the total annual funding is believed to run into millions of pounds. Earlier this year, the Commons' science committee recommended that the NHS should stop funding homeopathy on the grounds that it is a waste of money and it gives patients the false impression that such treatment works.

'When the NHS funds homeopathy, it endorses it. Since the NHS Constitution explicitly gives people the right to expect that decision on the funding of drugs and treatments are made "following proper consideration of the evidence", patients may reasonably form the view that homeopathy is an evidence-based treatment,' the select committee's report said.

In its response to the report, the Government said that it will keep the position on NHS funding under review. 'However, we believe that providing appropriate information for patients should ensure that they form their own views regarding homeopathy as an evidence-based treatment,' it said.

Scientists point out, however, that if patients are told clearly that there is no credible evidence to support homeopathic treatments, this may undermine the only benefit that homeopathy is likely to provide, namely the well-established 'placebo effect' where someone feels and gets better because they believe a treatment is working.

'Doctors are not allowed to prescribe an honest placebo, even if they think that is the best they can do for the patient. But they are allowed to prescribe a dishonest placebo by referring the patient to a homeopath,' said Professor David Colquhoun, a pharmacologist at University College London.

'Certainly you may feel better after the pill, because you were getting better anyway, or because of the placebo effect. That can't justify your doctor giving a pill that contains nothing whatsoever,' Professor Colquhoun said.

> 'Doctors are not allowed to prescribe an honest placebo, even if they think that is the best they can do for the patient. But they are allowed to prescribe a dishonest placebo by referring the patient to a homeopath'

'If there is no evidence that homeopathy works beyond the placebo effect, why does the Government pay for it? The answer given to that is "patient choice". I dare say the patient would cheer up if the NHS paid for a bottle of Chanel No 5,' he said.

Professor Edzard Ernst, a specialist in complementary medicine at the Peninsula Medical School in Exeter, said: 'If the Government is serious about putting patient choice over evidence, it not only displays a profound misunderstanding of both these issues but should then also give cream cakes to diabetics and cigarettes to someone with a lung disease.'

Evan Harris, a former Liberal Democrat MP who sat on the Science Select Committee when it carried out its inquiry, said that the decision to continue NHS funding homeopathy by the Government is not a good start for the Health Secretary Andrew Lansley.

THE INDEPENDENT

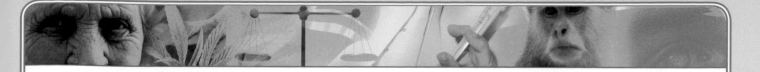

'How does the Government justify allowing treatments that do not work to be provided by the NHS in the name of choice, when it allows medicines which do work to be banned from NHS use?' Dr Harris said.

Homeopathy in numbers

⇨ **1796** The year in which a German physician called Samuel Hahnemann came up with the idea that 'like cures like'.

⇨ **£4m** Estimated amount spent on homeopathic treatments by the NHS each year.

⇨ **1,500** Approximate number of registered homeopaths in Britain.

⇨ **£150** Typical cost of an initial consultation with a homeopath.

⇨ **0%** Usual amount of active ingredient contained in each homeopathic remedy.

3 August 2010

© The Independent

No to homeopathy placebo

Using homeopathy on the basis that patients benefit from the placebo effect would be unethical and short-sighted.

By Edzard Ernst

When I began my research as Professor of Complementary Medicine in Exeter 17 years ago, I was entirely open to homeopathy. I had been treated for many years by a homeopathic doctor, my father had practised homeopathy and I had begun my medical career in a homeopathic hospital. But now my job was to apply science to the field and, to do this properly, one needs to be not just open but also critical.

The first thing any critical mind has to note is that the two basic assumptions of homeopathy fly in the face of science. Like does not cure like and diluting remedies *ad infinitum* does not render them stronger but weaker. But perhaps there was something entirely new and undiscovered here, the stuff of Nobel prizes that revolutionises our understanding of nature?

The acid test, I thought, was whether homeopathic remedies behave differently from placebos when submitted to clinical trials. So we conducted several trials and published many summaries of the studies done worldwide. The results were sobering. Today there are about 200 clinical trials and the totality of this evidence fails to show that homeopathic remedies work.

But what about patients' experience? What about my own experience as a patient and later as a clinician? In fact, tonnes of data shows that people get better after seeing a homeopath. This is why homeopaths are adamant that their treatments work. Can this wealth of experience be overruled by scientific evidence?

When one begins to analyse this contradiction rationally it very quickly dissolves into thin air. The empathic encounter with a homeopath, the expectation of the patient, the natural history of the disease and many other factors all provide ample explanation for the fact that patients can improve even when they receive placebos.

This leads to the vexatious question: what is wrong with giving placebos to patients as long as they help? The answer, I'm afraid, is a lot. This strategy would mean not telling the truth to patients and thus depriving them of fully informed consent. This paternalistic approach of years gone by is now considered unethical.

Also, placebo effects are unreliable and usually short-lived. Moreover, endorsing homeopathic placebos in this way would mean that people may use it for serious, treatable conditions. Furthermore, if we allow the homeopathic industry to sell placebos we should do the same for big pharmaceutical companies – and where would this take us? Crucially and somewhat paradoxically, we don't need a placebo to generate a placebo effect. If I give my headache patient an aspirin and do this, as all good doctors should, with empathy, time and understanding, the patient will benefit from a placebo effect plus the pharmacological effect of the aspirin. If I prescribe her a homeopathic remedy, I quite simply deprive her of the latter. It is difficult to argue that this approach would be in the interest of my patient.

What follows is straightforward: homeopathy is yet another beautiful theory destroyed by ugly facts.

22 February 2010

© Guardian News and Media Limited 2010

THE INDEPENDENT / THE GUARDIAN

Pulling apart the placebo

Does neuroscience hold the key to our understanding of how dummy medicines have a biological effect?

'You must know that the will is a powerful adjuvant of medicine' – Paracelsus (1493–1541), Swiss alchemist and physician.

Once, people with angina underwent surgery; small incisions were made in their chest and knots were tied in two arteries, to encourage blood flow to the heart. It seemed to work: nine out of ten patients reported improvements.

But in the 1960s, a young Seattle cardiologist, Leonard Cobb, ran an unusual clinical trial. He made the same chest incisions but left the arteries untouched. Remarkably, this 'sham surgery' was just as effective as artery knotting.

If placebos are beneficial, does it really matter if homeopathy has no specific benefits?

How can a treatment with no biological impact have a beneficial effect? This is the question Henry Beecher posed in his paper *The powerful placebo* in 1955, where he reported that an average of 32 per cent of patients across 26 studies responded to placebo, or dummy treatment. Some 50 years later, people are still trying to find out why.

Sugar is the pill

The placebo effect is an uncomfortable challenge to prevailing medical orthodoxy. Modern medicine sees disease predominantly as a disruption to body biochemistry; medicines are chemical entities that modify body biochemistry to restore health. By this model, sugar pills, say, should not have a physiological effect. But the evidence is unequivocal: they do.

Even more bizarrely, the nature of the placebo effect depends on the nature of the placebo. Red, yellow or orange pills provoke a strong stimulatory or antidepressant effect; blue, purple or green tablets are good for tranquilising reactions; and white pills are associated with analgesia – especially if they are seen to come from pharmaceutical packaging. Big tablets have stronger effects than smaller ones, and the more someone takes, the larger the effect.

This all suggests that expectations influence our response to medications. The idea that psychological factors affect conditions with a strong subjective element – such as pain or depression – may seem plausible, but can the power of thought really affect, say, heart function? The startling success of, for example, sham surgery suggests it can.

All in the mind?

So how might the placebo effect work? Recently, research has begun to reveal mechanisms of placebo action. In doing so it could provide valuable lessons for medicine.

One finding is that there are probably multiple placebo effects, not just one. For a start, some conditions spontaneously resolve, so treatment – real or placebo – actually had no impact. More interestingly, the placebo response can result from a learning process, a kind of conditioning. Having experience of receiving pain relief from a small, white aspirin may mean that taking a placebo similar in appearance could elicit the same effect.

The challenge for biomedical science is that placebo and treatment seem to belong in different realms – the 'mind' of the placebo effect with the 'matter' of body biochemistry. Recently, though, researchers have begun to reconcile mechanistic biomedical explanation with phenomenology.

'There's evidence of activation of chemicals in the brain when there's expectation of pain relief,' says Professor Jon-Kar Zubieta from the University of Michigan, who has used a brain-scanning technique (positron emission tomography) to show that expectation of analgesia activates the brain's own painkilling mechanisms.

The Michigan team looked at mu-opioid receptors, a class of receptors involved in endogenous pain relief. The activity of these receptors was higher when a 'painkilling' placebo was given with a painful stimulus, suggesting that the placebo stimulated the release of endogenous painkilling chemicals in the brain.[1] Consistent with this idea, a chemical that blocks the action of opioids in the brain prevents the analgesic effects of placebos.

Other work has shown that the degree to which someone anticipates relief can also affect the brain's responses. A US team has shown that certain brain areas associated with pain were activated less when subjects expected a lower level of pain. When subjects expected less pain they also reported lower pain scores.[2]

THE WELLCOME TRUST

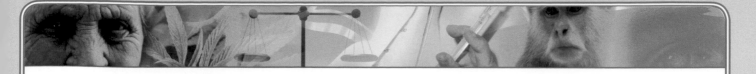

So, maybe there really is something in the saying 'mind over matter'? Professor Zubieta certainly thinks so. 'In many ways, how someone deals with pain is exactly mind over matter. What is unclear, however, is why some people can show this resilience to pain, and others not.'

In people with healthy brains, there is a marked difference in how individuals respond to placebo – a discrepancy that Professor Zubieta is keen to explore. 'The aim for us is to understand how people can learn to control these pathways. We anticipate that a number of factors affect this skill, and think that common genetic variants between people may be involved.'

Although pain has been particularly well studied, it is not the only condition affected by placebo responses. People with Parkinson's disease, for example, tend to respond well to placebo, and again the effects are mediated through the brain's biochemistry. When individuals with Parkinson's were given a placebo and told that it should improve their motor function, dopamine pathways (which are defective in Parkinson's) were activated and their arm movements improved.

Brain imaging has revealed that activation in several different brain areas is associated with placebo responses, including emotion-processing areas and the prefrontal cortex – the 'thinking area' of the brain.

But placebo effects are not restricted to the brain. Changes in brain activity can also influence other physiological functions – corresponding placebo effects have been noted on breathing and heart rate. Even the immune system can be modulated: after repeated associations between an immunosuppressor (cyclosporine A) and a flavoured drink, the drink alone can suppress immune system function.

The placebo in practice

The influence of the placebo effect in one field of medicine has been debated for many years: complementary and alternative medicine (CAM).

In a recent meta-analysis comparing 110 homeopathy studies with matched conventional medical studies, a team led by Professor Matthias Egger at the University of Berne, Switzerland, found that there was only weak evidence for an association between homeopathy and specific treatment effects, suggesting that homeopathy effectively works as a placebo.[3]

The report inevitably proved controversial. But if placebos are beneficial, does it really matter if homeopathy has no specific benefits? 'All medical treatments have non-specific effects,' points out Dr George Lewith, head of the Complementary Medicine Research Unit at the University of Southampton. 'The efficacy of many treatments is very small. For example, 80 per cent of patients with depression get better with a placebo.'

Moreover, adds Dr Lewith, 'Acupuncture, chiropractic and osteopathy all have specific effects.' It's just that these are very little studied.

Many doctors will admit to prescribing drugs that they don't think will work, or even sugar pills. And if a significant proportion of patients get better as a result, is this a problem? Might the placebo have a rightful place in the modern pharmacopoeia?

The difficulty is that the placebo response depends on an individual's belief – so use of a placebo depends on deception of a patient. Many question the ethics of this approach.

Professor Egger is among the sceptical. 'Giving a patient a placebo undermines your relationship with them. It's difficult to do as a doctor.' Instead he suggests that we learn from the approach adopted by CAM practitioners. 'Patients get better because people listen to them,' he says. 'In terms of homeopathy, practitioners often have more time to spend with their patients than GPs do. The shared belief of the practitioner and patient in the efficacy of the therapy is also very powerful.'

> ### 'Giving a patient a placebo undermines your relationship with them. It's difficult to do as a doctor'

There is a lesson here for modern medical practice, he adds. 'The whole-body approach should not be delegated to alternative medicine. Any good doctor should of course listen and consider the whole person. The distinction should not be between complementary and conventional medicine, but between interventions of proven effectiveness and interventions not supported by the evidence.'

References

1   Zubieta JK et al. Placebo effects mediated by endogenous opioid activity on mu-opioid receptors. *J Neurosci* 2005;25(34):7754–62.

2   Koyama T et al. The subjective experience of pain: where expectations become reality. *Proc Natl Acad Sci USA* 2005;102(36):12950–5.

3   Shang A et al. Are the clinical effects of homeopathy placebo effects? Comparative study of placebo-controlled trials of homoeopathy and allopathy. *Lancet* 2005;366(9487):726–32.

⇨ The above information is reprinted with kind permission from the Wellcome Trust. Visit www.wellcome.ac.uk for more information.

© *Wellcome Trust*

THE WELLCOME TRUST

WHO cares about the dangers of homeopathy?

The recent decision by the World Health Organization to advise against the use of homeopathy for serious diseases followed a campaign by young doctors and scientists who alerted the world to its tragic effects in developing countries. HealthWatch's president Nick Ross reports on this triumph of reason.

By Nick Ross, journalist and broadcaster

One of the criticisms of conventional, allopathic medicine is that it is dangerous. Indeed it is. It has been claimed that about 200,000 people die each year in the US as a result of preventable medical mistakes and infections which, if true, would be a higher toll than through road accidents[1]. Even more conservative estimates, of 44-88,000 deaths a year, puts healthcare risks on a par with bungee jumping and mountain climbing[2] (they all result in more than one death for every 1,000 encounters).

The UK figures are comparable, and three years ago the then Chief Medical Officer, Sir Liam Donaldson, reckoned: 'The evidence...from scheduled airlines is the risk of death is one in ten million. If you go into a hospital in the developed world, the risk of death from a medical error is one in 300.'[3]

These mishaps happen for many reasons, not least that patients often bring infections into hospitals and ill people tend to be especially vulnerable to hospital-acquired diseases, but there are also failings in diagnosis, prescription errors, unforeseen drug interactions and surgical mistakes. Clinicians are acutely aware of this and, particularly in the last decade, a great deal of emphasis has gone into improving systems to make things safer.

Alternative practitioners claim that what they do is less invasive and more 'natural' and so carries fewer risks; and to some extent, at least in theory, they are right. It is the very potency of allopathic medicine that makes it dangerous while, conversely, it is the impotence of most complementary therapies that can make them relatively safe. But folk medicine is not just anti-scientific, or at best pseudoscientific, with rarely any better outcomes than placebo. It too can be positively dangerous. Ray Tallis, the geriatrician and health ethicist, points out that the Mbeki Government's 'traditional' approach to AIDS in South Africa has led to over a third of a million unnecessary deaths. It is hard to compare numbers because, while proper healthcare systems have invested heavily in improving their audit of medical errors, the CAM community keeps few such records.

But some of the dangers are obvious, most notably misdiagnosis, which is far more likely with lay practitioners than with those who are medically qualified, and even more so at the hands of people who believe in pre-Enlightenment ideas about disease. Some of the treatments are also hazardous, including many herbal remedies (some of which have had to be outlawed), spinal manipulation, and even misplaced acupuncture needles. One of the most common generic traditional treatments, bloodletting, certainly killed far more people than it cured before it fell out of grace. Then there is the danger of downright crooks and charlatans who flourish amid the desperation of illness. (A friend of mine died from cancer having spent a great part of his family's savings on quack remedies.) But perhaps the greatest menace comes from the well-intended alternative practitioners. The danger is belief itself.

I, like many other HealthWatch supporters, became involved in this issue when I met women who had been offered 'alternative' treatments for cancer and had missed out on therapies that would probably have saved their lives and certainly could have prevented appalling suffering. In rural Africa and China I learned how primitive faith in traditional medicine effectively results in many diseases not being treated at all, with resulting disfigurement and miscarriages. But perhaps the most striking example of how 'natural' and 'safe' treatments can do harm is that of the most 'natural' and, ostensibly, the safest therapy of all. Homeopathy.

Homeopathy is simply water, adulterated only by a drop of credulity. How can that do harm? But the Voice of Young Science network realised it could, and did. The young medics (among them biochemist Evelyn Harvey who wrote for the last issue of the *HealthWatch Newsletter*[4]) cited examples of homeopathy being used as a preventative or as a therapy for a whole range of life-threatening conditions including HIV, TB, malaria, influenza and infant diarrhoea. And they have just won an important victory.

For many years the World Health Organization appeared to equivocate about the use of complementary medicines, and was sometimes cited by folk therapists as a justification for their practices. The WHO is a

HEALTHWATCH

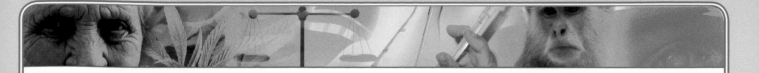

highly political organisation, subject to all sorts of governmental pressures and trying to juggle competing views of the world with the scientific realities of medicine and disease. It was easy to prevaricate in the hope of pleasing everyone. But in June the Voice of Young Science wrote to the WHO[5] and asked them to come off the fence. Specifically they asked the organisation to make it clear that people with conditions like HIV, TB and malaria should not rely on homeopathic treatments.[5] A few weeks later the WHO finally agreed.[6]

So it's now official. Homeopathy can kill, has probably killed thousands, and maybe tens of thousands round the planet. Now perhaps we should reflect on how astonishing it is that an ostensibly rational world could have thought anything different.

References

1   Harmon K. Deaths from avoidable medical error more than double in past decade, investigation shows. *Scientific American* 10 August 2009. View on http://www.scientificamerican.com/ blog/60-second-science/post.cfm?id=deaths-from-avoidable-medical-error-2009-08-10

2   Richard Smith, Reducing medical error and increasing patient safety. Presentation can be viewed on http://resources.bmj.com/files/talks/medicalerror.ppt

3   Sir Liam Donaldson, quoted in Hall S. Medical error death risk 1 in 300. The *Guardian* 7 November 2006. View on http://www.guardian.co.uk/society/2006/nov/07/health.lifeandhealth

4   Harvey E. Homeopathy and the developing world: dangers and lessons. *HealthWatch Newsletter* Jul 2009; 74: 1.

5   For details of the letter see http://www.senseaboutscience.org.uk/index.php/site/project/331/

6   For details of the response see http://www.senseaboutscience.org.uk/index.php/site/project/392/

October 2009

⇨ The above information is an extract from the HealthWatch newsletter and is reprinted with kind permission. Visit www.healthwatch-uk.org for more.

© HealthWatch

Mass homeopathy 'overdose' protest outside Boots

Members of the public who doubt the effectiveness of homeopathic remedies have held a mass 'overdose' protest outside Boots stores to make their point as part of the 10:23 campaign.

Supporters of Merseyside Skeptics Society (MSS) have urged high-street chemist Boots to stop stocking the remedies, claiming they are 'scientifically absurd'.

They gathered outside branches of the store in Liverpool, Manchester, Glasgow, Edinburgh, London, Leicester and Birmingham to swallow bottles of tablets.

Homeopathy tries to help the body heal itself, using very highly diluted substances.

Michael Marshall, from the MSS, said: 'We believe that they shouldn't be selling sugar pills to people who are sick. Homeopathy never works any better than a placebo. The remedies are diluted so much that there is nothing in them.'

He took a remedy said to contain arsenic but explained that the chances of finding one molecule of the substance in the tablets were incredibly small.

Mr Marshall said that consumers trust the company and it should not sell the remedies alongside mainstream medicines.

Similar demonstrations were planned in Canada, Spain, the US and Australia, he added.

The chief executive of the Society of Homeopaths, Paula Ross, said: 'This is an ill-advised publicity stunt in very poor taste, which does nothing to advance the scientific debate about how homeopathy actually works.'

1 February 2010

⇨ The above information is reprinted with kind permission from *Nursing Times*. Visit www.nursingtimes.net for more information.

© Nursing Times

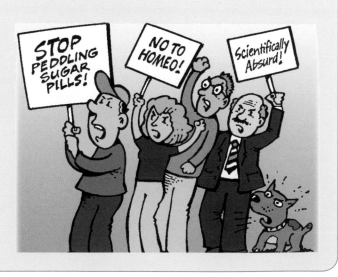

HEALTHWATCH / NURSING TIMES

The British Homeopathic Association dismisses 10:23 campaign

Information from the BHA.

The BHA regards the 10:23 stunt as grossly irresponsible. To suggest in public that taking an overdose of a medicine is a good way of testing its effectiveness gives an extremely dangerous message to the public. It also shows that the participants have no understanding about how to select and use homeopathic remedies in an appropriate manner.

> **To suggest in public that taking an overdose of a medicine is a good way of testing its effectiveness gives an extremely dangerous message to the public**

The claims of 10:23 ring hollow indeed. The evidence base for homeopathy is gradually increasing. There are well over 100 double blind trials in homeopathy and more are positive than negative. This is in spite of the many difficulties encountered squeezing a holistic and individualised treatment into a strictly controlled trial methodology.

Fascinatingly the evidence for the effectiveness of highly diluted substances in the laboratory setting is also mounting. Two commonly used models are the effect of highly diluted histamine on basophil activity and the effect of dilute arsenic on the growth of arsenic-impregnated wheat seedlings. These have been replicated by different groups of researchers. A full summary can be found in Dr Peter Fisher's submission to the House of Commons Science and Technology Committee. This whole field has been ignored by the critics of homeopathy as has the importance of patient outcomes.

The Faculty of Homeopathy and BHA do not support the sole use of homeopathy for any serious disease when effective conventional treatment is available to, and tolerated by, the individual patient. Homeopathy is, however, often used with great patient satisfaction for support during conventional treatments.

It would be a catastrophe if a small minority of cynics stifle patient choice of access to what they find effective. NHS patients have benefited greatly from homeopathic treatment – at a very small cost – with approximately £152,000 per annum spent on homeopathic medicines, which is a mere 0.001% of the NHS drug budget.

8 February 2010

⇨ The above information is reprinted with kind permission from the British Homeopathic Association. Visit www.britishhomeopathic.org for more information.

© British Homeopathic Association

BRITISH HOMEOPATHIC ASSOCIATION

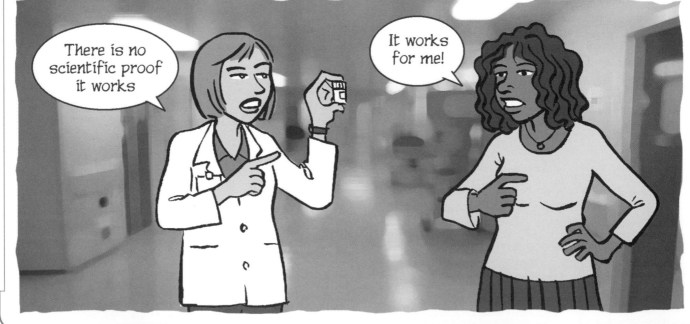

Herbal medicine is under threat

Alternative medicines face a backlash just when clinical research is turning back to nature.

By Bibi van der Zee

Tomorrow, an army of medical herbalists will be demonstrating outside the House of Commons. 'What are they going to do,' wonders sceptic Adam Rutherford, an editor at the science journal *Nature*, 'wave strands of lavender at MPs?' But Michael McIntyre, chair of the European Herbal and Traditional Medicine Practitioners Association (EHTPA), has called for the demonstration because, quite frankly, he has had enough.

For several decades, it's true, the field of complementary and alternative medicines (CAMs, as they are often known) has boomed, with acupuncturists, osteopaths and homeopaths springing up on every corner. Lately, however, a fierce backlash has been brewing. Scientists such as Professor Edzard Ernst (who puts complementary medicine's claims through clinical trials), and writers such as the *Guardian*'s own Ben Goldacre, have turned a long-needed microscope on to CAMs and accused them of being at best harmless, and at worst fraudulent and toxic. Herbal medicine was described by Rose Shapiro, in her book *Suckers: How Alternative Medicine Makes Fools Of Us All*, as mostly 'ineffective... if it worked and was safe it wouldn't need to be alternative... Herbal medicine should be subject to the same evidence-based regulation as are orthodox pharmaceuticals.'

These days, though, the majority of herbal practitioners are crying out for regulation, but despite promising to implement this for 20 years now, the Government is still dragging its heels. Meanwhile, discredited herbalists are able to continue practising, giving the field a bad name. And next year, when European legislation comes in which will stop unregulated practitioners from accessing many key herbal medicines, UK herbalists may well find themselves snookered.

But it has not all been bad news, as some new clinical trials have proved the efficacy of various herbal treatments. A review of studies of hawthorn (authored by Ernst) concluded that it is not only useful as a treatment for chronic heart failure, but also carries few of the risks associated with some conventional medicines. Horse chestnut, in another study by Ernst, has been shown to be useful for treating chronic venous insufficiency (when leg veins are not strong enough to pump blood back up to the heart), again with fewer side effects than conventional equivalents. And some of the studies on St John's wort have shown that it can improve symptoms of depression.

Garlic, another common herbal treatment, is regularly shown to reduce blood cholesterol, while black cohosh, an ancient Native American treatment, has had some success in clinical trials of its efficacy in treating menopausal symptoms. Studies of green tea, meanwhile, have shown that it can help inhibit tumour growth.

But this is not enough for the sceptics. 'Yes, a few herbal treatments may turn out to be medically effective,' says Rutherford. 'But for every one that turns out to work, there are hundreds that are just b******s. It's not half and half; many of these treatments turn out to be no better than a placebo.'

And yet scientists are increasingly turning back to the natural world in their search for modern medicines. Research is throwing up rich and intriguing results, showing that, among other things, the combination of tomatoes and broccoli is more effective in combatting tumours than either vegetable used alone; that cranberries really are effective at preventing urinary tract infections; that ginger can reduce nausea in the early stages of chemotherapy.

Declan Naughton, professor of biomolecular sciences at Kingston University, was part of a team which last year showed that mixing pomegranate rind with metal salts and vitamin C created an ointment effective at fighting the hospital superbug MRSA. 'As time has gone on,' he says, 'it has become more and more clear to me that a great number of the drugs we use originate from plants. If you were to sit down and list them, you'd be speaking for a long while, and if you're looking at developing new drugs, then you should obviously look to nature.'

Could there ever be a meeting of minds between ancient herbal and modern medics? 'You do have [herbal practitioners] following practices that are just unacceptable,' says Naughton. 'But you also have an increasing number of scientists screening herbs to find new drugs; more and more scientists are turning back to the original sources of medicine, the micro-bacteria, marine organisms and plants from the rainforests.'

'For centuries now we've been using these treatments,' says McIntyre, a herbalist himself for 30 years. 'It's profoundly frustrating to have to spend so much time battling to get ourselves regulated when what I'd really like to be doing is be in my practice, treating people.'

2 February 2010

© Guardian News and Media Limited 2010

THE GUARDIAN

Herbal medicines 'should be regulated'

Ipsos MORI report shows that 77% of adults agree that it is important that herbal medicines are regulated.

The Medicines and Healthcare products Regulatory Agency (MHRA) commissioned a programme of research by Ipsos MORI to identify the public's view on herbal medicines. The report sought opinion on safety issues arising from usage, the regulation of herbal products and how the public obtains information about herbal medicines. The research involved both quantitative surveys and discussion group discussions.

Historically, in the UK, most herbal medicines have been unlicensed. In 2005 the MHRA launched the new Traditional Herbal Registration Scheme (THR), which means herbal medicines now have to be made to assured standards of safety, quality and patient information. Companies with existing unlicensed herbal medicines on the market have until 2011 to register them with the Agency.

Richard Woodfield, Group Manager for Herbal Medicines at the MHRA, said: 'We welcome the findings of this research. The research shows that the public clearly see a need for herbal medicines to be regulated. So it is encouraging that the MHRA has already received 53 applications to register products under the THR scheme and that 25 products have so far been registered. However, we are not complacent and acknowledge that the research also shows that the MHRA has challenges ahead. Of recent users of herbal medicines (defined as those who have used a herbal medicine within the last two years), 58% agree with the statement that "herbal medicines are safe because they are natural". This means that the public still remains vulnerable to some of the less responsible operators who peddle low grade, and sometimes, dangerous herbal products – portraying them as natural and safe whilst failing to meet any meaningful standards of safety, quality and consumer information.'

Notes

Some key findings from the Ipsos MORI survey are shown below. For further information the Ipsos MORI report is on the MHRA website and also on the Ipsos MORI website.

General public usage of herbal medicines

⇨ 35% of adults have used a herbal medicine, and 26% of adults have used a herbal medicine in the past two years.

Usage of herbal medicines is higher among women and among those from higher social groups AB (higher or intermediate managerial, administrative or professional occupations), compared with men and those in lower social groups D and E (semi and unskilled manual workers and those on a state pension).

⇨ 77% of users of over-the-counter (OTC) herbal medicines have used an OTC herbal medicine within the past two years.

Perceptions of risk

⇨ 89% of respondents who have used herbal medicines in the last two years feel that most herbal medicines are safe to take.

⇨ 58% of respondents who have used herbal medicines in the past two years agree with the statement that 'herbal medicines are safe because they are natural'.

⇨ 67% of respondents who have used herbal medicines in the last two years agree that it is necessary to tell your GP if you are taking herbal medicine, while 22% of this group feel that telling your GP is not necessary.

Regulation

⇨ 29% of British adults believe herbal medicines are currently regulated in the UK, whereas 31% believe they are not and 30% don't know. The remaining 10% believe that some herbal medicines are regulated, and some are not.

⇨ 77% of adults agree it is important that herbal medicines are regulated, with this figure rising to 87% among regular users of herbal medicines (defined as those who have used a herbal medicine within the last two years).

⇨ Features of regulation that British adults feel are particularly important include: a check that ingredients are safe before the product is allowed to be sold (83% of all adults saying this is either 'essential' or 'very important'); a check that the manufacturer has quality controls to ensure the product contains what it says on the label and a leaflet explaining how to use the product and any likely side-effects (84% and 83% respectively saying that these are either 'essential' or 'very important').

Information

⇨ Doctors have been used as a source of information about the risks or benefits of herbal medicines by just under one in five (17%) of British adults. Relatively informal sources of information about herbal medicines are also widely used, as are pharmacists.

IPSOS MORI

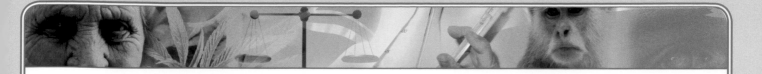

This includes family (15%), friends, colleagues and workmates (13%), pharmacists (9%), herbal or traditional medicine practitioners (8%), sales assistants in herbal medicine retail outlets (7%).

⇨ Sources that British adults are most likely to trust for accurate information about the risks and benefits of herbal medicines are doctors (41%) and pharmacists (23%).

The UK traditional herbal registration scheme was launched in 2005, which requires products to meet assured standards of safety, quality and patient information. There is a transitional period for some existing unlicensed products until 2011. Regulated products distinguished by their traditional herbal registration (THR) number on the packaging are progressively coming onto the UK market. As of December 2008 the MHRA had received 53 applications to register products under the scheme and had so far registered 25 products. There also continues to be available licensed herbal medicines, shown by the PL number, which meet MHRA-assured standards.

Historically, most over-the-counter herbal medicines in the UK have been sold as unlicensed herbal remedies under s12(2) of the Medicine Act 1968. This regime provided the public with little protection against low grade products. Repeated examples were found on the UK market of dangerous products, e.g. containing heavy metals, undeclared pharmaceutical substances or the wrong, toxic herb.

The MHRA is the government agency responsible for ensuring that medicines and medical devices work, and are acceptably safe. No product is risk-free. Underpinning all our work lie robust and fact-based judgements to ensure that the benefits to patients and the public justify the risks. We keep watch over medicines and devices, and take any necessary action to protect the public promptly if there is a problem. We encourage everyone – the public and healthcare professionals as well as the industry – to tell us about any problems with a medicine or medical device, so that we can investigate and take any necessary action. www.mhra.gov.uk

Technical details

This programme of research involved both qualitative and quantitative research among British adults. The details of each stage of the research project are as follows:

General Public Qualitative Research: four discussion groups were conducted between 8 and 10 July 2008 at two locations; one in the North (Stockport) and one in the South (Croydon) of England. Two groups were conducted in each location, one with users, and one with non-users of herbal medicines.

General Public Quantitative Research: Questions were placed on the Ipsos MORI Omnibus. A nationally representative quota sample of 2,305 adults (aged 15 and over) was interviewed in 197 sampling points throughout Great Britain. Interviews were carried out face-to-face in respondents' homes. Fieldwork was conducted between 5 and 11 September 2008. Data are weighted to match the profile of the Great Britain adult population.

12 January 2009

⇨ The above information is reprinted with kind permission from Ipsos MORI. Visit www.ipsos-mori.com for more information.

© Ipsos MORI

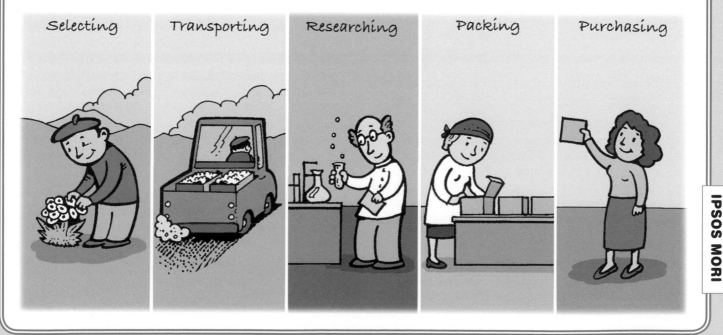

Selecting　　Transporting　　Researching　　Packing　　Purchasing

IPSOS MORI

Faith makes regulating herbal medicine difficult

A judge this week called for traditional medicine to be regulated, but it's not easy when practitioners make claims based on faith.

By Ben Goldacre

You may have read about Ying Wu this week: a traditional Chinese medicine doctor operating out of a shop in Chelmsford, Essex, who for several years prescribed pills with high doses of a dangerous substance to treat the acne of senior civil servant Patricia Booth, 58. Following this, her patient lost both kidneys, developed urinary tract cancer, had a heart attack, and is on dialysis three times a week. Judge Jeremy Roberts gave Ying a two-year conditional discharge, saying she could not be blamed, because she did not know the pills were harmful and the practice of traditional Chinese medicine is unregulated in Britain, a situation that he suggests should be remedied.

> **What worries me is that when you try to slot the square peg of faith-based medicine into the round hole of regulation and university teaching, you create more problems and confusion than you started with**

This sounds attractive, and has been welcomed by alternative therapists, who see regulation as the path to legitimacy. It's worth noting that we do already have systems in place for dealing with dangerous substances and people who prescribe treatments that have dangerous side-effects.

But regulation for alternative therapists raises a simple problem: it's hard to regulate practitioners who make claims based on faith. Attempts at regulation have exposed these contradictions. The Complementary and Natural Healthcare Council has a code of conduct that forbids alternative therapists making claims without evidence. Blogger Simon Perry complained about every reflexologist on the register on the day they joined if they were claiming to treat things such as arthritis, infertility, babies with colic and so on. All were told off, but the CNHC decided that fitness to practise was not impaired because the practitioners would have honestly believed their claims to be reasonable, since they would have been trained to believe they could treat these diseases.

So is training the problem? The Government's review into regulation of alternative therapists has recommended that it should be compulsory to have a university degree in alternative therapies, and that universities should run such courses. What is taught on these courses? You cannot know, because universities have gone to shameful lengths over many years to keep the contents of these science degrees a closely guarded secret.

Myself and Professor David Colquhoun of University College London have obtained course materials from students who thought they were going to be taught the scientific evidence base for alternative medicine, and have been dismayed by what they found. Handouts from the Bachelor of Science degree in Chinese medicine at Westminster University, for example, show students being taught – on a science degree – that the spleen is 'the root of post-heaven essence' and is responsible for the 'transformation of qi energy', 'keeping the muscles warm and firm'. We also see the traditional anti-vaccine spiel, as students are taught that vaccination is a significant cause of cancer.

A lecture by Niki Lawrence on 'Herbal approaches for patients with cancer', meanwhile, discusses the difficulties of the Cancer Act, which was specifically designed to protect patients from the more dangerous extremes of alternative therapists' self-belief. 'Legally you cannot claim to cure cancer' it begins, on a slide headed 'Cancer treatment and the law'. 'This is not a problem because: "we treat patients not diseases".' Lawrence then explains that poke root is 'especially valuable in the treatment of breast, throat and uterus cancer', *Thuja occidentalis* is 'indicated for cancers of possible viral origin, e.g. colon/rectal, uterine, breast, lung' and *Centella asiatica* 'inhibits the recurrence of cancer'.

It is a tragedy that someone has contracted a fatal condition and is on dialysis. What worries me is that when you try to slot the square peg of faith-based medicine into the round hole of regulation and university teaching, you create more problems and confusion than you started with.

20 February 2010

© *Guardian News and Media Limited 2010*

THE GUARDIAN

Advice to consumers: safe use of herbal medicines

Information from the Medicines and Healthcare products Regulatory Agency.

General advice to consumers

Remember that herbal remedies are medicines. As with any other medicine, you should use them with care while first ensuring they are the correct products for you. Also remember that the phrases 'natural', 'herbal' and 'derived from plants' do not necessarily mean 'safe'. Many plants can be poisonous to humans, and many pharmaceutical medicines have been developed from plants using the powerful compounds they contain.

⇨ Any medicine – herbal or otherwise – has the potential to have adverse effects (or side-effects).

⇨ Herbal medicines can also interact with other medicines you are taking. This could result in reduced or enhanced effects of the other medicines, including side effects. If you are consulting your doctor or pharmacist about your health or are about to have surgery or an operation, always tell them about any herbal medicines you are taking.

⇨ As with all medicines, keep herbal medicines out of the sight and reach of children.

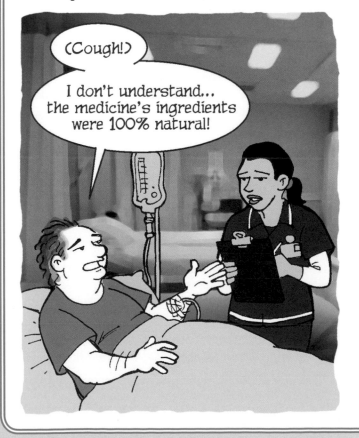

(Cough!)

I don't understand... the medicine's ingredients were 100% natural!

What you need to know as a consumer

Herbal medicines are medicines in their own right. As with any other medicine they are likely to have an effect on the body and should be used with care. The current weak regulation of herbal remedies in the UK has led to specific safety concerns which are also highlighted in this section.

> *Remember that the phrases 'natural', 'herbal' and 'derived from plants' do not necessarily mean 'safe'*

There are three possible regulatory routes by which a herbal medicine can reach you as a consumer. These are as:

⇨ Unlicensed herbal remedies. These products don't have to meet specific standards of safety and quality and so standards can vary widely. In addition, they are not required to be accompanied by the necessary information for you to use them safely, such as safety warnings and contraindications. Because this does not help the public to make informed choice or offer effective protection against low grade and dangerous products, by April 2011 all manufactured herbal medicines will be required to have either a traditional herbal registration or a product licence.

⇨ Registered traditional herbal medicines. A simplified registration scheme, the Traditional Herbal Medicines Registration Scheme, began on 30 October 2005. Products are required to meet specific standards of safety and quality and be accompanied by agreed indications, based on traditional usage, and information for the patients on the safe use of the product. Consumers can find general advice on the operation of the Traditional Herbal Medicines Registration Scheme within the herbal medicines pages of the MHRA website.

⇨ Licensed herbal medicines. Some herbal medicines in the UK hold a product licence or marketing authorisation just like any other medicine. These are required to demonstrate safety, quality and be accompanied by the necessary information for

MHRA

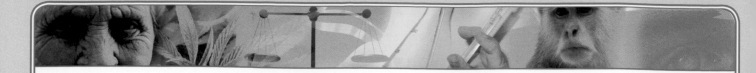

safe usage. These products can be identified by a distinctive nine-number Product Licence (PL) number on the product container or packaging which is prefixed by the letters PL.

Are any particular groups at risk?

The safety of many herbal medicines has not been established in certain key groups, including:

⇨ pregnant women;

⇨ breastfeeding mothers;

⇨ children;

⇨ the elderly.

All medicines, including herbal medicines, may cause side effects or unwanted reactions

Caution should therefore be taken when using herbal medicines, or giving them to someone else – particularly individuals in these groups.

⇨ As a rule, anyone with a history of liver or kidney complaints, or any other serious health condition, is advised not to take any herbal medicine without speaking to their doctor first.

Which herbal medicines have been assessed by government regulators (MHRA)?

In the Ipsos MORI report published in November 2008, 77% of adults agreed it is important that herbal medicines are regulated. Features of regulation that British adults feel are particularly important include a check that ingredients are safe before the product is allowed to be sold (83% of all adults saying this is either 'essential' or 'very important'). Some herbal medicines are indeed regulated by the MHRA, and meet assured safety standards. These are licensed and have a PL (or Product Licence) number on their labels. In 2005, the MHRA also launched a new registration scheme for herbal medicines – the Traditional Herbal Registration Scheme (THR) – under which herbal medicines have to be made to specific standards of safety and quality. These products have a THR number on their labels.

⇨ A herbal remedy without a PL or THR number on its label is unlicensed and has not been assessed by the MHRA, therefore nothing is known about its safety, quality, or any potential side-effects.

Companies with existing unlicensed herbal medicines on the market have to register them with the MHRA under the THR scheme by 2011.

It is not generally possible for consumers to identify which unlicensed medicines are made to acceptable standards. However, there are a number of pointers, in particular from the product information, which may be indicative of poor or unreliable standards.

How can I find out about the safety of individual herbs?

Once a herbal product has had its safety and the safety of its ingredients assessed by the MHRA, it will be given a licence with a PL or THR number. As unlicensed medicines have not had their safety checked, and information for the consumer may be patchy and incomplete, the MHRA has started a new service:

⇨ We are preparing information sheets on the safe use of individual herbs, which can be found under the herbal information sheets section of the MHRA website. The information will be based on herbal products that have been assessed since October 2005; this number will grow as more registrations are granted under the new THR scheme.

These information sheets aim to provide consumers with advice on specific herbal ingredients. This may help consumers identify, and avoid, any unlicensed herbal products which may come with unreliable or incomplete consumer information.

Remember that the quality, strength and usage of individual unlicensed herbal products may vary widely. This means that the MHRA information sheets can only be a broad guide to consumer information that should ideally be provided by the manufacturer of the product.

What to do if you think you have had an adverse reaction to your herbal medicine

All medicines, including herbal medicines, may cause side-effects or unwanted reactions. If you think you have had a reaction to your herbal medicine, you should discontinue using it and tell your doctor or pharmacist.

If you think you or someone else has had an unwanted or harmful reaction after taking a herbal medicine (commonly referred to as a suspected adverse drug reaction), we would like to know. This will help us give advice to other patients and healthcare professionals – and will help us make sure herbal medicines in the UK are safe.

⇨ You can report a reaction yourself directly to us using a system called the Yellow Card Scheme.

⇨ This can be done online at http://yellowcard.mhra. gov.uk/ or by filling out a paper yellow form which is available upon request by calling 020 7084 2000.

MHRA

⇨ Alternatively, you can ask your doctor or pharmacist to report the reaction to us on your behalf.

Any information received by us will be held in complete confidence and your personal details will not be given to anyone else without your permission.

Advice for consumers when buying unlicensed herbal medicines

Consumers should be alert and cautious when buying or using unlicensed herbal medicines. Any claims that a product is safe should be backed by credible evidence.

⇨ You should be wary of, and avoid, products making claims such as:

↳ The herbal remedy is '100% safe'.

↳ Herbal remedies are 'safe because they are natural'.

↳ This herbal medicine 'has no side-effects'.

↳ 'Chinese medicines will not interfere with the effects of any other medicine'.

↳ 'You can avoid Chinese medicines interfering with other medicines if you take them an hour apart'.

The MHRA strongly advises you not to follow any instructions for unlicensed medicines which state that you should stop taking, or change the dosage of, a prescribed medicine.

⇨ Always consult your doctor about making changes to your prescribed medication.

⇨ Treat with caution any unlicensed herbal medicine making claims that the product can prevent, treat or cure illnesses. These claims will not have been assessed by the MHRA and could be misleading.

⇨ Be wary of any product if it is not labelled in English, or if it does not have information about safe usage or a list of ingredients.

Unlicensed herbal medicines which are similar to each other may be accompanied by different patient information. Do not assume that the medicine with fewer warnings is necessarily safer to use.

Buying herbal medicines over the Internet

Again, the best advice for consumers when it comes to buying herbal medicines over the Internet is to be alert and cautious. There is an international trade in poor-quality, unregulated and unlicensed herbal products. Some of these have been found to contain banned pharmaceutical ingredients or heavy metals which are poisonous. Products may also contain harmful herbs that are not permitted in the UK, and you should be aware that unlicensed herbal medicines manufactured outside the UK may not be subject to any form of effective regulation.

⇨ Even if a product has been granted a licence in another country, there may be no guarantee that it complies with the requirements and standards of UK-regulated products.

22 April 2010

⇨ The above information is reprinted with kind permission from the Medicines and Healthcare products Regulatory Agency. Visit their website at www.mhra.gov.uk for more information on this and other related topics.

© MHRA

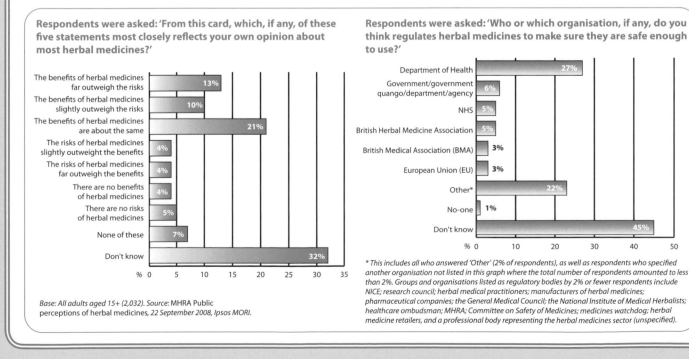

Respondents were asked: 'From this card, which, if any, of these five statements most closely reflects your own opinion about most herbal medicines?'

- The benefits of herbal medicines far outweigh the risks — 13%
- The benefits of herbal medicines slightly outweigh the risks — 10%
- The benefits of herbal medicines are about the same — 21%
- The risks of herbal medicines slightly outweight the benefits — 4%
- The risks of herbal medicines far outweigh the benefits — 4%
- There are no benefits of herbal medicines — 4%
- There are no risks of herbal medicines — 5%
- None of these — 7%
- Don't know — 32%

% 0   5   10   15   20   25   30   35

Base: All adults aged 15+ (2,032). Source: MHRA Public perceptions of herbal medicines, 22 September 2008, Ipsos MORI.

Respondents were asked: 'Who or which organisation, if any, do you think regulates herbal medicines to make sure they are safe enough to use?'

- Department of Health — 27%
- Government/government quango/department/agency — 6%
- NHS — 5%
- British Herbal Medicine Association — 5%
- British Medical Association (BMA) — 3%
- European Union (EU) — 3%
- Other* — 22%
- No-one — 1%
- Don't know — 45%

% 0   10   20   30   40   50

* This includes all who answered 'Other' (2% of respondents), as well as respondents who specified another organisation not listed in this graph where the total number of respondents amounted to less than 2%. Groups and organisations listed as regulatory bodies by 2% or fewer respondents include NICE; research council; herbal medical practitioners; manufacturers of herbal medicines; pharmaceutical companies; the General Medical Council; the National Institute of Medical Herbalists; healthcare ombudsman; MHRA; Committee on Safety of Medicines; medicines watchdog; herbal medicine retailers, and a professional body representing the herbal medicines sector (unspecified).

MHRA

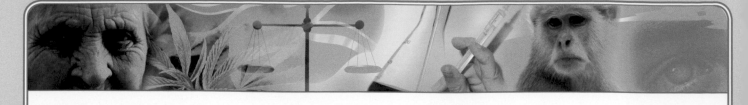

KEY FACTS

⇨ More and more health professionals such as doctors, nurses and physiotherapists use various kinds of complementary and alternative medicine (CAM). (page 1)

⇨ In many cases the risks associated with complementary and alternative therapies are associated more with the therapist than the therapy – for instance a trained acupuncturist would never reuse needles, and a trained herbalist will be aware of the possible risks. (page 2)

⇨ A report in the *Lancet* in 2007 stated that about 13,000 patients were treated at the five (now four) homeopathic hospitals in the UK each year. 14.5% of the population say that they trust homeopathy and £38 million is spent on homeopathy each year in the UK. (page 3)

⇨ Another reason why patients may choose complementary and alternative medicine is that they receive more time, empathy and emotional support from an alternative therapist. There may also be a spiritual component that they like. (page 5)

⇨ In the UK, up to one-third of people with cancer (33%) use some sort of complementary therapy at some time during their illness. For some types of cancer, such as breast cancer, the number of people using complementary therapies is even higher at almost half (50%). (page 6)

⇨ Although many complementary therapies are 'natural', it doesn't necessarily mean they can't cause harm. Some herbal remedies may cause side effects or interfere with conventional treatments. (page 7)

⇨ Only 2% of UK consumers currently buy most of their medicines or healthcare treatments online. (page 8)

⇨ Herbal medicine is among the most ancient forms of treatment known and the medicinal use of plants is common to all cultures and peoples of the world. (page 10)

⇨ NHS herbal medicine is now available, in a very limited capacity, and much also depends on a doctor's view of complementary therapies. (page 11)

⇨ All herbal medicines sold over the counter in the UK should according to the law be licensed. The MHRA assesses them on safety, quality and patient information. By 2011 a new scheme, which is currently being rolled out, will be in place. (page 13)

⇨ Medics at a BMA conference voted overwhelmingly in favour of banning homeopathic remedies being funded by the NHS and withdrawing backing for the UK's four homeopathic hospitals. (page 16)

⇨ As well as around 400 GPs who integrate homeopathy into their practice in the UK, there are four NHS homeopathic hospitals – Bristol, Liverpool, London and Glasgow. (page 18)

⇨ Last year, the *Guardian* newspaper reported that the NHS spent £12m on homeopathy from 2005-08. The Society of Homeopaths estimates that £4m is spent annually. (page 20)

⇨ Homeopaths believe that homeopathy can help with any condition that the body has the potential to repair itself. (page 25)

⇨ 1,500 is the approximate number of registered homeopaths in Britain. £150 is the typical cost of an initial consultation with a homeopath. 0% is the usual amount of active ingredient contained in each homeopathic remedy. (page 27)

⇨ 89% of respondents who have used herbal medicines in the last two years feel that most herbal medicines are safe to take. (page 34)

⇨ 77% of adults agree it is important that herbal medicines are regulated, with this figure rising to 87% among regular users of herbal medicines (defined as those who have used a herbal medicine within the last two years). (page 34)

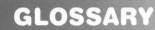

10:23 campaign

The 10:23 campaign consists of a group of people who are sceptical about the claims of homeopaths, particularly with regard to the efficacy of their products. In January 2010, members of the group took part in a demonstration outside the Boots chain of chemists, during which they took a massive overdose of Boots-stocked homeopathic remedies in order to show that they had no effect on health. Although the group claimed the protest was a success, the British Homeopathic Association condemned it as 'irresponsible'.

Acupuncture

An ancient practice which involves inserting sterile needles into strategic points on the human body with the aim of relieving pain and other negative symptoms.

Aromatherapy

Aromatherapy utilises scented 'essential oils', which practitioners claim will induce certain moods or promote good health.

Chiropractic

Chiropractors are practitioners of complementary medicine, and are legally-recognised professionals just like doctors and nurses. Chiropractic teaches that spinal disorders can affect the health of the body generally, and seeks to treat these through a combination of methods, including spinal adjustment and manipulation; massage; exercises, and lifestyle counselling.

Complementary and Alternative Medicine (CAM)

CAM includes a wide range of therapies and practices that are outside the mainstream of medicine: for example, homeopathy, herbal remedies, acupuncture, reflexology, reiki and traditional Chinese medicine. Complementary medicine uses therapies that work alongside conventional medicine. Alternative medicine includes treatments that are not currently considered part of evidence-based Western medicine. However, as the distinction between the two is not clear-cut, the term complementary and alternative medicine (CAM) is now widely used to include both approaches. The effectiveness of some forms of CAM is often hotly debated.

Homeopathy

A form of alternative medicine in which practitioners use highly diluted substances to treat their patients. The thinking behind this practice is that when substances known to cause certain symptoms are delivered to patients exhibiting those same symptoms in a highly diluted form, the substances will be effective as a treatment. According to the Society of Homeopaths' website, a homeopathic remedy of 30C contains less than one part per million of the original substance. While practitioners and patients are vocal supporters of the benefits of homeopathy, its critics claim that there is a lack of scientific and clinical evidence to support it and that it offers little more than a placebo effect.

Holism

A Greek word meaning 'all' or 'whole'. Holistic health teaches that an individual should be considered as a whole and offered medical treatments as such: hence the oft-cited CAM principle that complementary and alternative therapies treats the individual, not the disease. In alternative medicine, a holistic approach will take all of an individual's needs – physical, psychological, spiritual and social – into account when considering the causes of an illness and the best way to treat it.

Osteopathy

Osteopaths are practitioners of complementary medicine, and are legally-recognised professionals just like doctors and nurses. Osteopathic principles teach that treating bones, muscles and joints can aid the body in repairing itself.

Placebo

A placebo is a substance administered to patients containing no active ingredients: for example, a sugar pill or saline solution. However, the patient taking the placebo is led to believe that it is a medicine which will have a positive effect on certain symptoms they are displaying. The 'placebo effect' refers to an improvement in symptoms brought about by a patient's belief that the inactive substance they are taking will cure or improve their illness. Critics of certain types of alternative medicine, for example homeopathy, believe that the treatments given to patients by practitioners are little more than placebos.

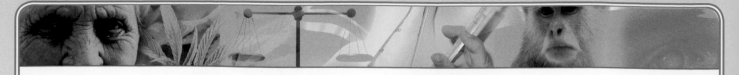

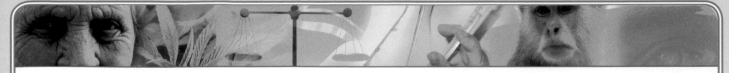

Additional Resources

Other Issues titles

If you are interested in researching further some of the issues raised in *Alternative Medicine,* you may like to read the following titles in the *Issues* series:

⇨ Vol. 197 *Living with Disability* (ISBN 978 1 86168 557 5)

⇨ Vol. 190 *Coping with Depression* (ISBN 978 1 86168 541 4)

⇨ Vol. 187 *Health and the State* (ISBN 978 1 86168 528 5)

⇨ Vol. 176 *Health Issues for Young People* (ISBN 978 1 86168 500 1)

⇨ Vol. 159 *An Ageing Population* (ISBN 978 1 86168 452 3)

⇨ Vol. 141 *Mental Health* (ISBN 978 1 86168 407 3)

⇨ Vol. 138 *A Genetically Modified Future?* (ISBN 978 1 86168 390 8)

⇨ Vol. 134 *Customers and Consumerism* (ISBN 978 1 86168 386 1)

⇨ Vol. 88 *Food and Nutrition* (ISBN 978 1 86168 289 5)

For a complete list of available *Issues* titles, please visit our website: www.independence.co.uk/shop

Useful organisations

You may find the websites of the following organisations useful for further research:

⇨ **Arthritis Research UK:** www.arthritisresearchuk. org

⇨ **British Homeopathic Association:** www. britishhomeopathic.org

⇨ **Cancer Research UK:** www.cancerhelp.org.uk

⇨ **European Herbal and Traditional Medicine Practitioners Association:** http://ehtpa.eu

⇨ **HealthWatch:** www.healthwatch-uk.org

⇨ **The King's Fund:** www.kingsfund.org.uk

⇨ **MHRA:** www.mhra.gov.uk

⇨ **NHS Choices:** www.nhs.uk

⇨ **Nursing Times:** www.nursingtimes.net

⇨ **Prince's Fund for Integrated Health:** www.fih. org.uk

⇨ **TheSite:** www.thesite.org

⇨ **Wellcome Trust:** www.wellcome.ac.uk

⇨ **World Health Organization:** www.who.int

⇨ **YouGov:** www.yougov.com

For more book information, visit our website...

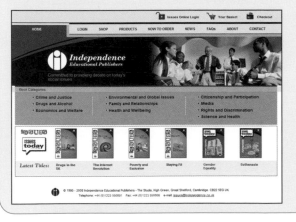

www.independence.co.uk

Information available online includes:

✓ Detailed descriptions of titles

✓ Tables of contents

✓ Facts and figures

✓ Online ordering facilities

✓ Log-in page for Issues Online (an Internet resource available free to Firm Order Issues subscribers – ask your librarian to find out if this service is available to you)

ACKNOWLEDGEMENTS

The publisher is grateful for permission to reproduce the following material.

While every care has been taken to trace and acknowledge copyright, the publisher tenders its apology for any accidental infringement or where copyright has proved untraceable. The publisher would be pleased to come to a suitable arrangement in any such case with the rightful owner.

Chapter One: Complementary Therapies

An introduction to complementary therapy, © Arthritis Research UK, *Complementary and alternative medicine,* © EMIS 2010 as distributed at www.patient.co.uk/doctor/Alternative-and-Holistic-Medicine.htm, used with permission, *Why people use complementary or alternative therapies,* © Cancer Research UK, *What words or phrases come to mind when I say 'herbal medicines'? [graph],* © Ipsos MORI, *Alternative antidotes,* © YouGov, *Traditional medicine: definitions,* © World Health Organization, *Herbal and traditional medicine,* © European Herbal and Traditional Medicine Practitioners Association, *Herbal medicine,* © TheSite. org, *Just how safe are herbal medicines?,* © Telegraph Media Group Limited 2010, *Call for more research into complementary therapies,* © The King's Fund.

Chapter Two: The Debate

Complementary medicine: health risk or the real heal?, © Telegraph Media Group Limited 2010, *BMA votes against homeopathy funding,* © Nursing Times, *EU to fund complementary medicine research,* © Prince's Fund for Integrated Health, *Supporters of homeopathy outraged at medical union's attacks,* © British Homeopathic Association, *An overview of NHS homeopathy,* © British Homeopathic Association, *Beliefs about herbal medicines [graphs],* © Ipsos MORI, *Ban homeopathy on NHS, say MPs,* © Channel 4, *Types of herbal medicines used [graph],* © Ipsos MORI, *Homeopathy works and is an important part of the NHS,* © British Homeopathic Association, *Government urged to embrace integrated health care,* © ePolitix, *Homeopathy remains on NHS,* © Crown copyright is reproduced with the permission of Her Majesty's Stationery Office – nhs.uk 2010, *Government ignored our advice on homeopathic remedies, say experts,* © The Independent, *No to homeopathy placebo,* © Guardian News and Media Limited 2010, *Pulling apart the placebo,* © Wellcome Trust, *WHO cares about the dangers of homeopathy?,* © HealthWatch, *Mass homeopathy 'overdose' protest outside Boots,* © Nursing Times, *The British Homeopathic Association dismisses 10:23 campaign,* © British Homeopathic Association, *Herbal medicine is under threat,* © Guardian News and Media Limited 2010, *Herbal medicines 'should be regulated',* © Ipsos MORI, *Faith makes regulating herbal medicine difficult,* © Guardian News and Media Limited 2010, *Advice to consumers: safe use of herbal medicines,* © MHRA, *Do the benefits of herbal medicines outweigh the risks?, Who regulates herbal medicines? [graphs],* © Ipsos MORI.

Illustrations

Pages 2, 10, 17, 22: Simon Kneebone; pages 6, 14, 20, 32, 37: Angelo Madrid; pages 8, 12, 18, 31, 35: Don Hatcher.

Cover photography

Left: © Toronox. Centre: © tinpalace. Right: © dcarson924.

Additional acknowledgements

Research by Mark Anslow.

And with thanks to the Independence team: Mary Chapman, Sandra Dennis and Jan Sunderland.

Lisa Firth
Cambridge
September, 2010